Care *of the* Ancient Ones

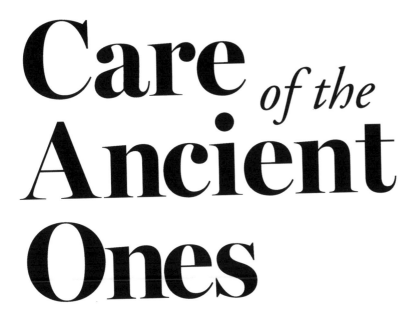

Care *of the* Ancient Ones

Gentle Eldercare in the
Rough-and-Tumble World
of Modern Medicine

Judith Murphy Millar
NURSE PRACTITIONER

ISBN-13: 978-0692715529
ISBN-10: 0692715525

Cover and book design: Claire MacMaster | barefoot art graphic design
Copy editor: Renée Nicholls
Cover image: Walker with Cane, istock

*Dedicated to my long-gone grandparents,
my first and still favorite, Ancient Ones.*

Contents

Preface

Our modern culture has evolved to create a whole new way of growing old. Shifting demographic trends reflect a rapidly growing population of older people. In 1900 there were only about three million people over the age of sixty-five in this country and less than 125,000 people who had survived to over eighty-five years old; at that time the average life expectancy was only forty-seven years. In stark contrast, recent projections indicate that there will be approximately eighty million people over the age of sixty-five by the year 2050. Sixty-five years is no longer even thought of as old.

Today, in the United States there are more than five million people over the age of eighty-five, and they are growing older every day. The oldest of the old are growing at the most rapid rate, with a 300 percent increase in the over-eighty-five population since 1960.

The "Ancient Ones" who are the focus of this book are not the young-old or the middle-old. They are the old-old, often ninety years or more, and they have varying abilities to care for themselves. The vast majority of them have at least some level of dependence on others due to medical, functional, or cognitive problems.

As well as the "old-old," younger individuals who have had a prolonged course of chronic illness frequently experience an accelerated aging process. They can be thought of as "Ancient Ones" at a much younger age. Conditions such as diabetes, chronic obstructive pulmonary disease (COPD), advanced cancer, heart disease, neurodegenerative diseases such as Parkinson's disease, multiple sclerosis (MS), Alzheimer's disease, other dementia-related illnesses, and some psychiatric disorders are some of the causes of premature aging.

Improved medical care, better nutrition, and a higher standard of living have allowed us to grow older and older. Many elders are now living with a constellation of chronic diseases that require medication and ongoing monitoring. Families are often geographically spread out, and caring for a frail elder from a distance can be a constant source of worry. Those living nearby commonly supervise or assist their elderly relative with a variety of tasks. Watching someone you care about grow frail, then frailer still, is challenging and often produces anxiety. It is never easy to know when to step in to help and when to back off to allow more autonomy. There is help available in most communities, but first we need to be able to recognize the Ancient One's needs and gain access to these services. The information outlined in this book is meant to provide general guidelines and a framework for readers to consider in the day-to-day realities of life as they weave a safety net for their beloved elders.

We all want our elders to be spared from unnecessary suffering, yet it can be hard to reconcile this desire with the attitudes and demands of the patients and their families. In many cases, it is possible to prolong life with medical treatment, but at the same time it is impossible to give that life any real quality.

During times of worsening status or even just failing to improve, patients and their families may ask questions such as "Can't you do something?" and "Why won't you do something?" These questions often reflect their false perception that providers have total power over illness; or they may suspect that information or treatment is being withheld for some reason. At other times, they may be concerned that some providers just don't care, act like they're too busy, seem inattentive, or are merely disinterested. Sadly, in some cases, they are right.

Our society is now faced with the task of providing elders with a safe and dignified lifestyle and meeting their healthcare needs, while spending healthcare dollars wisely and avoiding futile care. Healthcare providers want to make sensible and appropriate decisions that are consistent with their patient's wishes; however, in order to ensure that this occurs, they need to know what those wishes are.

A dilemma is occurring both on an individual level with elders in crisis and on a community level with gaps between the multitude of needs and the limitations of resources available for elders. As people age, their lives usually do not get easier. Previously healthy and independent people now need help. These changes can happen slowly over time or they can happen quickly in response to an acute medical event. The aging patient may need help for a brief time or a prolonged duration, even indefinitely. Currently it is estimated by the U.S. Census Bureau that approximately 70 percent of those over eighty-five have some sort of disability—including sensory, cognitive, or functional impairments—that requires the assistance of another person. Not surprisingly, up to half of people need physical assistance and this increases dramatically with advancing age.

I am a nurse practitioner. For over twenty-five years I have cared for generations of elders in the same skilled nursing facilities in Cape Ann, Massachusetts. My new patients come from the hospital and are at a crossroads in their health, ready for hospital discharge but not well enough for home.

While at the skilled nursing facility, the patient will interact with an interdisciplinary team involving numerous participants, and I will refer to that "team" often in these pages.

This team will establish both short- and long-term goals for the patient, as well as an individualized treatment plan to focus on his or her relevant issues. This plan of care will include services that vary in type, duration, and frequency, depending on the specific medical, nursing, or rehabilitation care these individuals need, along with their insurance coverage.

In my work, I spend a great deal of time with patients, their family members, and the healthcare team trying to come up with a safe plan for these frail elders. I find that having clear goals is the most important part of the plan. This book, which is based on my professional practice, personal experience, and ongoing study, is a primer for readers who are caring for the very old. It is about goals, approaches, and issues that impact the health and life of this growing population. Both family caregivers and healthcare professionals will find the perspectives in these pages useful when making a plan to keep elders safe, comfortable, and functional for as long as possible. Each chapter offers

- explanations of the important issues that affect the health and well-being of the very old;

- reality-based case studies to illustrate these issues in daily life;

- practical suggestions for managing an elder's complex physical and medical needs; and

- guidance to help readers address the difficult decisions that arise along the way.

The care of these frail and ancient folks is a daunting challenge. This book is not intended to be a substitute for appropriate individualized medical diagnosis or treatment. However, it *will* help you understand the issues, formulate a plan, and manage this crucial task. Let's get started.

Acknowledgments

This book has been a long, challenging, and difficult project—much like the job of providing elder care. Geriatrics, specifically the care of the very old, has long been a poorly regarded specialty practice. Not much glamour here, no fancy procedures, no miracle cures. The work is hard and reflects so much loss and decline. In spite of this, I have had the pleasure of meeting countless wonderful people who start as patients and—along with their friends and families—end as friends. I live in a great place. I meet interesting people every day. Thanks to these folks who teach me something every day.

The staff members and professional colleagues with whom I work are a great combination of lifelong residents, modern healthcare nomads, and immigrants from all over the world. We work together, trying to rise to the challenge of providing quality, dignified care in a highly regulated, paperwork-fixated, ever-changing healthcare environment. As one of my favorite doctors would say on his way out the door, "Thank you for all your good work."

I want to thank several people who helped me along the way. Joe Millar did a great early edit and his friend Ellen Bass was kind enough to give me wonderful advice. I did my best to take their suggestions. Renée Nicholls, my writing coach and editor, was invaluable and did several rounds of review. I'm not sure I could have done it without her assistance and encouragement. Olivia Gale, my research assistant, did what I did not want to. Thanks to Claire MacMaster for her encouragement and making this such a good-looking book. To my family and friends who endured my angst over this project, sorry and thanks. And those who knew nothing of this project, I wonder if you are surprised. Finally, a big thanks to my wonderful husband and daughter, Harry and Claire Millar. I finally finished!

Introduction

The following stories describe two elders who were doing quite well in spite of their advanced years—until a minor mishap occurred and set them back significantly. The first story involves a beloved grandmother.

Grandma and the Saturday Night Bath

It was a routine thing: Grandma's daughter, Joyce, stopped by the house every evening, and she phoned every morning to check that all was well. Nothing was unusual on Saturday evening when she left the house. However, that Sunday morning, the phone just kept ringing and ringing. Repeated attempts to call also received no response. Finally, as the phone continued to ring, Joyce tried to rationalize through the possibilities, visualizing the scenarios and not liking any of them. Grandma had a Lifeline emergency call button, which she was meant to push to notify responders in a crisis, but she was prone to taking it off and leaving it on the bedside table. Her daughter tried not to panic as she called her sister Beth and asked her to meet at Grandma's house.

Beth and Joyce arrived at the same time. They banged at the locked screen door but were answered by silence. They had a key to the main door, but they had to break through the locked screen door first. Finally, they were in. From the bathroom, a weak kitten voice called, "In here." Grandma was ninety- three, shivering, and in the tub, cold water faucet dripping. For sixteen hours she had struggled to get out, never giving up, never settling in with a towel to wait for morning. An ambulance was summoned to take her to the emergency room.

Luckily, Grandma had no major injuries; she was stiff, sore, and slightly dehydrated, which was easily remedied with a liter or two of IV fluids. She also had some skin breakdown on her bottom, called a decubitus ulcer, from the pressure of the hard tub on her soft body. She was home by the end of the day.

This was a wake-up call for both Grandma and her family. Up to that point, she had been so independent and steady on her feet, she had never fallen or experienced any mobility problems. She had taken a bath in that tub nearly every week for sixty years. It wasn't ever really clear why she couldn't get up on that night, but it was evident that she was changing and needed help. A week before it would have been hard to convince her of that necessity, but after her long, hard night she realized she was no longer as independent and capable as she once had been. She was truly frightened by her experience and therefore more open to accepting some changes in her routine.

Grandma was lucky she didn't get injured badly and was able to go directly home from the emergency room. On the other hand, she looked ten years older than the night before her ordeal, and she suddenly needed help getting up from bed. A few days later, after connecting with Grandma's doctor, Joyce was able to arrange for some home care. They had all just entered a whole new world.

As Grandma's story shows, we can identify two hurdles that existed even before this situation. First, Grandma was reluctant to have any home help prior to her fall. She had always insisted that she'd do just fine on her own. Second, the preventative plan that was in place—the emergency call button—had its own set of limitations. In many cases, and for many reasons, it is sometimes only possible to make life-saving modifications after a big event. This was also the case with Stanley.

Stanley

Stanley was an eighty-nine-year-old married, talkative astronomer. His wife suffered from dementia and lived on the Alzheimer's unit of a nursing home, and he lived alone with no nearby family. Up to this point he had been managing his affairs quite well and had recently traveled across the country on his own. However, his wife's caregivers were now concerned about his memory. He frequently asked repetitive questions, and he had started to miss some of his usual visiting times.

One day in January, a deliveryman pulled in to Stanley's driveway and noticed a car with its interior light on and the door opened. He parked the truck and called out. No one responded. Then he saw the feet. They were poking out from the snow bank. Soon he found a very cold man. Stan was moving but groggy. The deliveryman called an ambulance, and somehow managed to get him in the warm truck until the paramedics came and brought him to the hospital.

In the emergency room, doctors found that Stanley had a wound and a badly infected leg. He was admitted to the hospital for the required IV antibiotics. He also was suffering from dehydration, gastritis, and anemia. Further tests showed that he had experienced a minor heart attack, and had worsening of his existing kidney disease. He needed bed rest, wound care, and IV antibiotics for at least one week. Due to the level of care required, he was transferred to a skilled nursing facility for the continuation of the plan of care.

No one was ever sure what had happened to him, because he couldn't remember recent events. At the nursing facility, the healthcare team guessed that it all may have been started by a small cut on the back of his knee that he couldn't reach or even see. Perhaps when it became infected and started to hurt, he thought it was arthritis and took some over-the-counter pain medications—maybe several. Soon his symptoms likely included a little nausea and poor appetite, but at that time he had no awareness of the seriousness of his symptoms. Just as his problems were coming too quickly to manage, he decided to go for a drive . . . .

Stanley's hospital stay was complicated by periods of confusion and anxiety. He needed frequent reorientation regarding his medical problems and their treatment. He was particularly forgetful about his mobility restrictions, such as no walking, and nurses found him out of bed on many occasions. Fortunately, as his medical condition improved, his cognition did also, but he still had big gaps in his recent memory. His physical therapy progressed, although he continued to show poor safety awareness.

Stan wanted to go home immediately and lacked the insight to see why his family, who were consulted by phone from their home several states away, and his medical team were worried. However, he agreed to stay a few more days to give everyone time to try to sort things out.

Stanley's situation, like grandma's, shows that even a highly functioning elder is vulnerable. Like most elders at a rehabilitation facility, his goal was to return home to his independent life.

In Stanley's case, a "family and team meeting" was held to consider the social supports that existed in Stanley's life prior to his illness and to determine how to improve his home situation. Stanley had always been so capable, and the family had needed to devote so much energy to the sad decline of his wife, that there had been little consideration of his needs. The family now realized they had underestimated his aging difficulties and how little they knew of his medical issues. They made arrangements for Stanley to receive some help at home, particularly with driving, shopping, housework, and personal care. Everyone—including Stanley—finally recognized that the safety net needed to be cast farther out. When he returned home, he would still maintain independence, but he would now have regular contact with helpers who would come into his home and thus be able to keep an eye on him and report any changes.

* * *

Through my role as a nurse practitioner, I often meet patients in situations very similar to the ones faced by Grandma and Stanley. They may have been placed at our facility for their first short-term rehab stay or their tenth. They have been sick or hurt, or have had surgery resulting in debilitation. Some are "sharp as a tack" and highly functional, some are a little forgetful, others are totally confused, and many are somewhere in between. Like Stanley, most want to recover, get rehabbed, and go home. Many do. Some stay for long-term custodial care. Those who go home do so with a plan for home care services.

Remaining at home, or returning home, often depends upon the availability of both formal and informal services. Paid assistance, either privately financed or subsidized help, is the formal care. Informal help occurs when a willing friend or family member in the home or nearby volunteers to provide some assistance. Current statistics estimate that there are twenty million to fifty million informal caregivers, unpaid family, or friends in this role today. These devoted but largely unskilled caregivers are extremely important players in the health management of the elderly, providing up to 80 percent of that home care. The services they provide include shopping, laundry, home and finance management, transportation, personal care, medication monitoring, and many types of nursing procedures. When an elder is living alone, without a nearby support system, the challenges are much more difficult.

As I work with the patients, their family members, and the healthcare team to create plans for treatment, whether at home or in a facility, I find that it helps to identify any barriers to achieving the goal and to identify measurements that will indicate how well the team is staying on track. Of course, there are many courses of action and reaction for every medical situation, and I do not claim to know the best answer in these cases. (In fact, quite often there is no single correct answer.) There are, however, many questions that need be asked for each proposed course of action. The main ones are these:

- What are we trying to accomplish with this course of action?
- Is this course of action likely to create an outcome closer to or further away from our goal?

Thoughtful questioning can prompt a useful dialogue among the patients, their representatives, and healthcare teams. Conversations can be very time-consuming (especially when things haven't gone as planned), and teams may need to revise goals as patients either progress or do not. However, by establishing goals promptly and clearly, the team can simplify everyday decisions (for example, they can ask, "Does this decision bring us closer to our goal?") and help make these trying times easier for everyone involved.

Ideally, families and patients should discuss important topics such as safety and independence, comfort and function, and end of life issues far in advance of need. Along the way, they should work with the medical team to identify healthcare goals and arrive at an agreement on the approach to meet these goals. It's wise for elders to select a healthcare agent (and an alternate); healthcare agents are usually friends or family members who are entrusted to make important decisions in the event that the elders are not able to do so themselves.

Holistic and compressive plans of care are what keep elders engaged in positive lifestyle and healthcare practices. Specifically, care planning, as described in this book, will help readers and their families identify issues that define the problem and need attention. Disease processes and/or functional decline associated with chronic illness, such as heart or lung disease or dementia, usually result in predictable issues that threaten the elder's ability to manage and cope with the complex health problems. These issues frequently cross diagnostic and specialist lines and can often be best addressed with a practical approach and common sense. Consequently, learning about these potential problems will help readers and their families with consideration and planning and increase their chance to achieve the elder's healthcare and lifestyle goals, whatever they may be.

In an attempt to organize concepts that are not linear and have overlapping issues, I begin with the concept of goals of care and different approaches of achieving them. Chapter 1 discusses "The Plan," which includes both short- and long-term goals, with explanations about advance directives for life-sustaining treatments. Chapter 2 continues the plan, while identifying common approaches toward medical care (Life Is Good; Find It, Fix It; Never Say

Die; Know the Unknown; Father Knows Best; Live Free or Die; Don't Ask, Don't Tell; Care and Comfort). I discuss the pros and cons of each approach and include real-life scenarios to help readers identify and choose an approach to care that supports the elders' goals and helps families make wise decisions.

The middle portion of this book deals with issues of care primarily occurring in the home setting. Practical information provided in Chapter 3, "Home Sweet Home," includes a description of the challenges and obstacles to daily life as well as strategies for safety and independence. The goal for this time in life is to have a well-functioning plan in place, and the focus is on helping the elder stay well and at home.

The important activities of daily living (ADLs) that must occur in order for the elder to remain at home are discussed in Chapter 4. Basic self-care tasks like dressing, bathing, and toileting are covered here, along with more complex tasks such as meal planning and preparation.

In Chapter 5, "Accessing the Healthcare System" discusses the importance of communication between caregivers and healthcare teams and provides a "who's who" list of professionals that ancient ones and their families are likely to encounter.

The next three chapters deal with changing conditions as more problems develop. Chapter 6, "Trouble Brewing," offers key questions to help caregivers assess the elder's physical and mental condition. It also provides essential information about the four steps involved with most medical evaluations: identification of complaint, symptoms, and signs; evaluation; diagnosis; and treatment. This chapter covers medication orders and monitoring and also discusses various life-sustaining treatments. Chapter 7 covers basic physical issues that are common with ancient ones. These include issues with cognition, swallowing, heart and lungs, elimination, fluid balance, and pain. This practical perspective helps to simplify complex interactions between multiple concurrent disease processes. Chapter 8, "Care Where?" takes a look at places where some of these issues may be treated, ranging from community hospitals to nursing homes. It also offers tips for choosing the right nursing home should the time come when that level of care is required.

The final portion of the book deals with the more emotional and cognitive aspects of advanced age. Chapter 9 describes the common mental illnesses in the very old, their presentations, and discussion of management strategies, treatments, and side effects. Dementia and cognitive decline is the focus of Chapter 10. To help readers understand the stages of dementia easily, I compare them to stages of childhood: teen, preschool, toddler, and infant. I explain the challenges and provide strategies for dealing with the changing presentations of this difficult condition. In compassionate terms, Chapter 11 includes practical guidance for recognizing the subtle changes at end of life and how to prepare and care for the physical realities of dying. Lastly, a glossary is included at the end of the book to briefly explain unfamiliar terms.

* * *

For the families of the Ancient Ones, it can be a daily struggle to figure out "what the heck is going on" with their elderly relatives and how to help them. Every day I see families coping with these issues. Whether there is a major problem at hand or a sense of impending disaster, there is a bewildering array of social, functional, and medical matters to consider. The information described in this book will help readers sort out the most pressing concerns, provide a context or framework for the decisions at hand, and make a plan.

The stories in this book, which are based on the experiences of so many of the patients I've had the honor to work with over the years, will frame the issues, goals, and approaches toward healthcare decision-making. There is much we can learn from the stories of these ancient ones and their journeys through the last part of their long, long lives.

Chapter One

Make a Plan:
Establishing Goals of Care

The *plan*, which we will discuss throughout this book, refers to the individual's healthcare, including the issues involved and the decisions that need to be made.

From a medical perspective, the plan starts with the goals of care. Specifically, it is very important to identify what we are trying to accomplish with our interventions. When dealing with the very old, it is essential to appreciate the unique needs of this special population. This next section discusses common goals, both long- and short-term. To begin, let's look at the story of Iris to see what sort of plan needed to be made and how it needed to be updated as her situation changed.

Iris

Iris at ninety-four was a vibrant and highly talented working pianist, fully engaged in life. She played in church and at weddings, she gave lessons, and she had friends from multiple generations. Music was her life. Her spirit kept her active despite the fact that she had suffered all her life from severe spinal scoliosis and in later years with osteoporosis and arthritis. Her body grew shorter and more twisted every year. Thirty-minute swimming sessions released her from the burden of gravity, and she felt it was a gift. However, walking was a chore, particularly as her unsteadiness progressed. Observers winced as they watched her hobble around, and they prayed each time she got behind the wheel of the car.

Iris adamantly maintained her independence, resisting help or suggestions about simplifying her routine and improving safety. However, her falls became more frequent, and she became less skilled at covering them up. She still climbed stairs at home. Her family was concerned that she had hit her head a time or two—perhaps more—and she was not remembering things as she once did. When she ended up in the hospital for an infection in her leg, she was found to have widespread discolorations in several stages of bruise evolution, suggesting a series of unreported falls.

During the acute phase of her infection, some confusion washed through her but then passed. At rehab she was alert; oriented to person, place, and time; and pleasant and talkative. During the assessment of her case, the rehabilitation team discussed her goals and the issues surrounding them. Iris herself was very clear: she wanted to go home as soon as possible. She had things to do and didn't want to bother with inpatient physical therapy.

With that in mind, her family and the staff agreed that her current status of "home alone" could no longer be recommended. A major change would be required to achieve her goal of "safety at home." She would need to be willing to accept that others would have to do some things for her, and that meant moving her bed downstairs, at least until she was stronger.

Iris seemed to resign herself to these ideas. She didn't like the thought of being "babysat," but she reluctantly agreed.

Iris remained at the rehabilitation facility while plans were put in place to care for her at home. At the facility, she did very well for a few days and even participated with therapy, but the bumps and bruises of days gone by eventually caught up with her. She was stiff and sore. Unable to sleep or even rest, she was very uncomfortable. Mild pain medications were ordered to try to lessen the pain. One morning she didn't wake up. She was alive but minimally responsive. She looked gravely ill, though peaceful.

At this point, the staff and her friends and family needed to reconsider her goal of care—independence—which was no longer an option. What plan should be set in place in the absence of this goal? Working together, they recalled that during recent conversations with the healthcare team, Iris had expressed her long-term wish that, in the absence of the possibility of independence, she wanted her caregivers to avoid futile care and instead focus on comfort. She did not want any steps taken that would prolong a life of frailty and loss of independence.

Because Iris had stated her wishes clearly, the family was able to use them to guide the course of events that followed. In a situation like this, "care and comfort" is both a goal and an approach. We kept her where she was and did some simple bedside x-rays, blood tests, and urine tests, but found nothing specific to treat. She roused briefly, spoke to her daughters, lived for about a week as family and friends gathered at her bedside, and then peacefully died.

Iris's situation shows the need to consider both long- and short-term goals when making a plan for care. In this case, it was easy to define such a plan because she had shared her wishes with friends and family. Even though her short-term goals could not be met, her long-term goals of immediate care and comfort versus extended intervention were achieved, and that was very meaningful to her family. They were comforted by the knowledge that her end-of-life situation was so well directed.

When we consider the broad picture of life, what do most people want? Most people want the same things. Even people of vastly different circumstances have the same physical needs, and they want to have them met. Air, food, fluids, the ability to eliminate waste, shelter, rest, and activity are very basic physical needs that, if not met, will lead to sickness, decline, and/or death.

Only when these basic needs are satisfied can we move on to the not-so-clear-cut needs. We want to be happy, safe, and mobile, functioning well in our environments. Our society also values autonomy and independence. Self-determination encourages us to have control over as many aspects of our life as we can. Adults want to make their own decisions, or they want to choose to delegate others to make the decisions for them. Maintaining connections with family and friends is important to most people.

Regarding healthcare, we want to live a long, healthy life. We want to feel good—to be functional and free of pain and other uncomfortable or unpleasant symptoms. When sickness comes, we want early diagnosis and prompt, tolerable, and affordable treatments for disease. We want clear advice on how to modify our lifestyles to promote our well-being. When it becomes evident that end of life is near, we want to be told all necessary information so we can plan for our death with our families and healthcare providers.

The delivery of healthcare would be much easier if these assumptions were truly universal beliefs. Instead, it often seems that unrealistic expectations, hidden agendas, unhealthy relationships, and patterns of "bad habits" cloud and complicate the issues relating to health and healthcare. There are those for whom dependence and family manipulation are part of their daily activity. These are the people for whom illness or debility has some emotional value.

They receive increased attention from family members and declarations of love and pledges of loyalty that may make the "sick role" an overall pleasing experience. This can be a problem when healthcare providers, patients, or family members make the assumption that goals are mutual and that everyone is on the same page.

Oftentimes for the very old, any medical illness or injury can result in generalized weakness with a decline in self-care capabilities. This type of weakness will often be more prolonged than the precipitating illness and may or may not be entirely reversible. There is often waxing and waning of medical symptoms and associated functioning as these two areas interface. The elderly person's functional performance will fluctuate within a range of comfort and capability.

This is the "good days and bad days" phenomenon. On the good days it may seem there is excessive oversight, with the temptation to cut back on the help available. On the bad days there may never be enough help. With this phenomenon, it is important to budget care for the lowest level of function in order to maintain safety on the bad days.

In my work, I see people struggle with the issues of autonomy, safety, and mobility. Most know what they want, and their primary goal is to remain in their home or return there. But when their health takes a turn for the worse through sickness or functional decline, they must make some sort of change.

So what happens when these primary needs are not independently met? We need a plan. This plan must

1. identify the elders' personal goals, including basic and not-so-basic needs;

2. compare those needs with their ability to meet them;

3. determine the issues and where the deficits are; and

4. formulate the strategies and steps for corrective action, with the aim of meeting those goals.

As the stories throughout this book show, physical, functional, or cognitive impairments can preclude an elder's much-desired independence. Therefore, individuals need a plan that reflects their actual health and functional status and develops a reasonable approach toward their goals.

Unfortunately, some people have goals that are based exclusively on a sense of entitlement and confuse the "best" care with the "most" care. For instance, some families assume that the best setting for a frail elder is a major teaching hospital because any number of doctors, specialists, residents, interns, and students will be involved in the care. Patients and their families tend to expect that the teaching hospitals will use all the resources available in all indicated cases. The truth, however, is that while a great deal of medical information can be gleaned in this way, it often occurs at great physical and psychic expense to the patient and frequently results in very little gain in the quality of life. In such a case, is the goal of the "best" care met?

Many times the best care for a frail elder (especially those with a "care and comfort" goal) is to continue with their existing providers. Known providers are sometimes just exactly the best medicine. A local well-equipped hospital may easily handle the situation; in such cases it is not necessary to forfeit this setting—which is likely familiar and, as such, comforting to the patient—for the "best" care.

Other types of goals involve supporting the family as a whole, rather than the patient only. These include steps to lessen the "burden," which may be

- emotional (e.g., worry, anxiety, insomnia, resentment);
- financial (e.g., money spent on medicines, equipment or supplies, staff, and/or loss of assets or income from missed work);
- physical (e.g., labor for personal care or household chores); and
- time-consuming (e.g., managing finances, medical appointments, errands).

Preserving the family financial treasure may be a collective goal, or the ability to bequeath fortune may be of paramount importance. These goals may be clearly spoken, or they may be obscured by years of intergenerational fog. Some people are better than others at dealing with burden.

The first step to achieving goals of any sort is simply to identify them. In the next section, we'll take a look at some of the short-term goals that need to be met when caring for ancient ones.

Short-Term Goals: Where Do We Go from Here?

During initial assessments, the team will determine both short-term and long-term goals as the first part of care planning. Short-term goals address the immediate problems at hand. For instance, let's say that an elderly woman who is experiencing weakness due to an infection falls, breaks an ankle, and gets admitted to the hospital. In this case, the primary goals—and the first order of business—involve medical stabilization (treating the infection and repairing the bone) as well as symptom management. This is done at the hospital, where it is determined that she cannot be directly discharged home.

At this point she is transferred to a skilled nursing facility for further care. There, the next immediate short-term goal is to address functional issues, promoting comfort, mobility, and independence. During the rehab stay, other issues may be addressed, such as cognitive decline, depression, or any number of important concerns. As well, the staff may help the patient and her family evaluate and improve the formal and informal support system at home. This all goes hand in hand with a discharge plan.

Whenever a timeline is proposed for a plan, there will always be the question of how long it will take for the elder to get better. There is no other answer than "it depends." The success of any one plan of care will depend upon a great number of variables, including

- the condition of the patient before the most recent medical event;
- the severity of the illness;
- the number of days spent in bed;
- the number of complications; and
- the severity of any of any setbacks (which can always be expected).

These issues show why we need a back-up plan as well as an overall approach. We must continue to consider all of these issues as we go forward with the plan toward the identified goal. Part of the plan will include anticipating complications and trying to prevent or minimize the problems.

Arranging for support services to ensure a safe transition to home is another part of the plan. This often leads to the big question: After rehab, can Mom go home again or is another living situation needed?

The return-to-home (or stay-at-home) plan is a reality for those who are able to meet their own needs or are able to have their needs met with the help of either formal or informal caregivers. If the challenges of independent living are limited to housekeeping, shopping, meal preparation, and bookkeeping, this is an easier fix with delegation to informal support or formal services. It is a much harder problem if there is insufficient strength, endurance, or balance for independent safe movement in and out of bed and to and from the bathroom and kitchen. In this case, modifying the living space or adding adaptive equipment may improve these problems.

If the assistance of one person for transfers and personal care is sufficient, then a home care arrangement may be a reasonable plan. The care at home becomes much more difficult when the assistance of two helpers is needed due to severe disability or weakness. This is often a situation when nursing home placement becomes necessary.

Unfortunately, cognitive decline can create problems that no pill, device, or equipment can remedy. This situation requires another person to be on hand to provide assistance. In such cases, when the elder either lives alone or with someone who is unable to provide the required amount of assistance, it may be necessary to consider alternative living situations. The individual's options vary depending upon the specific circumstances. Elders in this situation may move in with family; choose elderly housing, assisted living, or a nursing home; or try adult foster care or congregate living.

Long-Term Goals: Advance Directives

While it may seem odd to talk about long-term goals for people who are already fifteen years—or more!—beyond the average life expectancy, a discussion of the topics covered in this section should not be put off. The long-term goals I am referring to involve determining what is wanted and not wanted at the very end of life, as well as how to proceed with anticipated decline. Advance directives help ensure that those wishes are carried out should the person be unable to communicate them to the medical healthcare team.

Even though I believe most people in this age group have a very practical attitude toward end-of-life decisions, this is a better discussion to have with a healthy person than a sick one. In this section, I am only going to discuss these topics in a general or philosophical way. In later chapters I will provide the more nitty-gritty details of medical care during the elder's last days.

HEALTHCARE AGENTS AND ADVOCATES

Adults who are sound in mind and body are presumed to be competent to make their own decisions, even bad ones. These decisions don't have to be popular, nor do they require consensus or approval.

As noted earlier, a healthcare agent is a person—usually a family member or friend—whom elders appoint to make decisions should they not be capable of doing so themselves. In fact, sometimes an elderly person who still is capable opts out of the decision-making process and puts the designee in charge. (This is considered temporary but may in fact become the case over and over again.) The job of the healthcare agent is to make decisions on behalf of the patient—decisions that the patients would make themselves if they were able. As part of their responsibility to the patient's wishes and intentions, healthcare agents (also called *proxies*) should never implement their own preferences.

In the absence of a designated proxy, decisions may need to be settled by the legal system, with a family member or friend petitioning to be the proxy or in some cases with a guardian appointed by the court. Laws about the legal process as well as the rights and responsibilities of healthcare agents and guardians will vary from state to state.

Medical care requires consent, and decisions need to be made. The more serious or complicated the problem, the more decisions need to be made. Inpatient facilities require patients or their healthcare agents to sign a "consent to treat" form that gives permission for routine medical care. It is always advisable to ask what is considered "routine care," as it varies. Specialized treatments, procedures, or surgeries require a specific consent form. In skilled nursing facilities, psychoactive medications require their own consent form.

When there is a medical situation and the patient is unable to understand the issues or make decisions, then the healthcare agent is asked to step up to the plate. In most cases, there will first be a medical and/or psychiatric evaluation to determine the patient's thinking and communication status. When it is clear that the patient lacks the capacity to comprehend the situation, the healthcare agent is invoked or activated by the medical healthcare team. At this point the designee or agent is asked to make decisions and sign consents.

The designation of a healthcare agent is the first and most basic step toward creating a long-term plan for care. All adults should complete a *healthcare proxy*, a simple form that can be completed in the healthcare or other setting. It does not require a lawyer. This step is particularly crucial for those of advanced age or with a serious medical or mental illness diagnosis.

The specific terminology for these documents and roles vary from state to state. It is important to include alternate agents, since the spouses and even children of the very old may also be elderly. Although this document does not have an expiration date, it can be changed at any time. If there is more than one, then the most recently dated form is the one that is valid.

Before we move on, let's take a quick look at Hilda's story, which shows how quickly a plan can run off course if the healthcare agent does *not* speak up to convey the patient's wishes—even (and perhaps especially) in cases where certain types of treatment are considered "standard" or "routine care" and no further consent or consultation with the patient or agent is required.

Hilda

Hilda was a ninety-four-year-old delightful Finnish widow from out of town who came under my care. She had problems of memory loss and poor judgment. Prior to her decline she had appointed friends to serve as her healthcare agent (and an alternate) if a time came when she was not capable of making her own decisions. They had little awareness of her past medical history but knew her overall life philosophy.

Recently hospitalized for the treatment of mild heart failure, Hilda was too weak to go back to her most recent home—an assisted living facility that specialized in caring for those with dementia—and the hospital doctor believed she would benefit from rehab. In terms of personal goals, although she might not remember the date or who the president was, she knew enough to state that she wanted to return to the assisted living facility she called home. She had a Do Not Resuscitate (DNR) order. Her friends supported the plan for her to return there.

While at rehab she developed shortness of breath, and on two occasions she was sent to the emergency room. There was a rapid resolution of the symptoms with simple measures but no clear diagnosis. The doctor decided to run more tests. She had trouble holding still for the testing and a pulmonary emboli (blood clot in the lung) could not be definitively ruled out. She was prescribed anticoagulants (blood thinners) just in case. The blood thinners caused internal bleeding and anemia. Then she suffered a heart attack. Throughout this time, her healthcare agent did not participate or question any of the doctor's decisions, which were made primarily to cover the legalities of the situation (that is, to avoid the legal risk of not treating the potentially life-threatening possibility of a blood clot). Ultimately, Hilda recovered and was well enough to return to her assisted living, but in the end she was weakened more by the medical care than by her original presenting symptoms.

In this case, the patient's short-term goal had been to return to assisted living. She also had the long-term goal of DNR. Although Hilda was too demented to comprehend the benefits and risks associated with any particular treatment, it was well acknowledged by her friends that she wanted to avoid institutionalization more than she wanted to avoid death. The intention was that all treatment would be aimed at helping her achieve the goal of returning "home" as quickly as possible. However, the addition of anticoagulants tipped the safety scale in the wrong direction. Healthcare providers didn't consider her personal goals as much as the medical legal risks associated with omitting treatment for a potentially fatal event. *This whole plan occurred with the inaccurate presumption of shared goals*, which might have been avoided had the healthcare agent spoken up for Hilda and discussed with the doctor the pros and cons of evaluation of symptoms and treatment in terms of Hilda's goals and wishes.

In summary, Hilda's story is an example of someone with the foresight to appoint local friends as healthcare agents, to whom she expressed her goals (although not her medical details, which I also recommend). However, her goals were put aside by the medical team, who took steps to fix a potential problem she very likely would have chosen not to treat. At this time, her healthcare agent did not speak up on her behalf. Consequently, during the detour away from her goal, she received treatment for a problem not clearly present, and she suffered serious complications that were both painful and debilitating. These treatments actually prolonged her recovery and rehab; meanwhile, the tests remained inconclusive.

Part of the reason that Hilda's care was confusing was that even though she had identified a healthcare agent, this person was chosen because she was a friend and not because she was medically oriented, assertive, or curious. When the time came for her to act, she was a bit uneasy with her role and was not sure what she was meant to do. Questioning "doctor's orders" was not on her mind. She did not serve as an *advocate*.

In fact, whether patients have a healthcare agent or not, it is advisable to have a trustworthy and capable advocate to help ensure that any issues don't fall through the system's cracks. Specifically, whether the elderly patient is incapable of making decisions or not, the advocate can act as a support person to

- help keep track of the details;

- keep a journal when things get complicated;

- attend care-planning meetings;

- ask questions; and

- help listen to medical updates.

Often this is the healthcare agent. Other times it may be a different family member, neighbor, or friend who is more readily available to be physically present and then communicates with the official decision-maker (agent).

LIVING WILLS

Advance directives also involve the personal beliefs behind the issues. Living wills are a type of document that basically states that the individual accepts that death is part of life and has no desire to participate in medical care that is considered to be futile. Living wills are a legal document with powers that vary by state, and they are frequently completed with a lawyer.

Living wills are useful when patients can no longer speak for themselves and suffer from a terminal condition. Common phrases in these documents focus on the hope that the patient's life will not be prolonged through "extraordinary medical intervention" if there is no hope for a "meaningful recovery." Some documents are very explicit about how doctors come to the conclusions about what is a "terminal condition."

It's important to note that these documents may not always be used in an emergency or urgent situation when decisions need to be made quickly and bulky terminology is more subject to interpretation. Therefore, even with a living will, if the patient has a cardiac arrest, CPR may be performed if there is not yet a documented "terminal condition" and there may be "a chance" for meaningful recovery.

LIFE SUPPORT DIRECTIVES

Many states now have a version of Medical Orders for Life-Sustaining Treatments (MOLST) or, in some states, Physician Orders for Life-Sustaining Treatments (POLST). This is a state-by-state initiative that provides an actual medical order for the use or non-use of specific interventions considered to be life sustaining. These include CPR, intubation and mechanical ventilation, feeding tubes, dialysis, and intravenous treatments for hydration. There is also the choice that allows "do not transfer to hospital except for comfort."

This final option serves as an official mechanism to allow gentle eldercare, including end-of-life care, in their current setting whether this is their family residence or a nursing home. This is a new and important option that had been long absent. It provides support for the great number of people who want a peaceful death but otherwise would be whisked off to the hospital for an "episode" or change in condition that "might" evolve into an end-of-life situation. The truth is that many of these episodes are recurrent, and with an individualized treatment plan for comfort, ancient ones can often be easily treated in their own familiar place with simple measures.

As noted, these forms are relatively new and show great potential for implementing patients' wishes. No diagnosis of terminal illness is needed, and healthy people of advanced age can protect themselves from unwanted life-sustaining medical care. The MOLST may be updated or changed as the patient's situation or status changes.

These wishes are translated to actionable medical orders and move from setting to setting with the patients. This means, for example, that if individuals have an active DNR on the MOLST form, that same document can go with them from home, to the emergency department, to the hospital room, to the skilled nursing facility. This replaces the cumbersome process of needing to obtain a new order—or worse, forgetting to obtain one—for each new healthcare setting.

* * *

There is no one document or plan that is perfect and will cover every possibility, but these forms are so much better than nothing. Discuss the options with healthcare providers to get your questions answered.

As noted earlier, the very most important way to ensure that wishes are honored in the event of incapacitation is to choose the healthcare agent wisely. Choose someone (and at least one backup) who will be able to deal with stress and emotional conflict and who will be readily available, especially if there will be need for ongoing contact between the healthcare agent and the medical team. Complete the required forms and then keep copies in the medical record, the lawyer's office, and in the "important papers" place in the home.

Earlier we looked at Hilda's case to see what can happen when the healthcare agent does not step up to the plate. Now let's take a moment to look at what may occur in the sudden event of a serious illness when there are no advance directives in place (or they are not readily available), the medical team proceeds with multiple tests and treatments, and the family isn't sure what to do.

Mr. Nash

At ninety-two, Mr. Nash was slowing down. He was keeping to himself, slowly disengaging from life. He was slightly confused and seemed apathetic, but not unhappy, sleeping his days away. When he just picked at his food and lost weight, his worried wife brought him for a physical, but he had no specific complaint for the doctor, other than being tired and achy. The blood work was fine and he checked out okay on the physical exam. He was diagnosed with mild depression and early dementia. Then, just as these issues were starting to stabilize, he had a stroke.

His wife returned from the morning shopping and found him slumped in the chair. He was breathing but unresponsive and she called 911. Mr. Nash was admitted to the hospital with a massive stroke, which resulted in complete paralysis of the right side of his body, an inability to swallow anything at all, and very limited speaking ability. He was hospitalized for a few days and then transferred to rehab for continuing care. Hydration was maintained with an IV for about ten days to wait for any return of neurological function. This didn't happen. During this time he became weaker without any nutrition, while the family tried to come to grips with this new situation.

He was alert enough to sustain the briefest of conversations, but due to the severity of the stroke, he was unable to understand and couldn't be expected to make any thoughtful decisions related to his care. His vocabulary seemed to be limited to just a few words, and the medical team suspected that his words may not have matched his thoughts because of aphasia, the loss of ability to understand or express speech, caused by brain damage. He was nearly immobile and could not sit up without support or swallow any form of fluids or nourishment.

A decision needed to be made, but there were no advance directives in place to state his wishes for treatment, and his family was not sure what to do. Even though death is a natural consequence of such a massive stroke, the family did not want to let him starve to death (as they perceived it), so they agreed to have a feeding tube inserted through his skin into his stomach. This provided a route for hydration, nourishment, and medication. Once these basic needs were met, his nutrition improved but not his strength or mental capabilities.

As time went by, in spite of ongoing physical rehab, Mr. Nash had no functional gains. He continued to require total care and had little ability to communicate. After just a few weeks he developed a painful skin breakdown, requiring frequent dressing changes and pain meds. Soon the feeding tube was causing difficulties of its own, and he became uncomfortably intolerant to it. He was miserable. He experienced persistent pneumonia, as well as abdominal distention with constipation and diarrhea, which soiled his bedsores. Because of all the problems, the healthcare team needed to reduce the feeding rate, but that caused a new dilemma because this decreased rate of feeding was neither keeping him nourished (his family's goal) nor comfortable. Clearly, none of this made any sense.

After a family and team meeting, the plan changed. Comfort measures were instituted, with tube feedings discontinued. Mr. Nash died in a few days. In the end, his family recognized that his dying was far easier to witness than what had become of his life.

In contrast, Edith's final days were quite different from Mr. Nash's because she did have advance directives in place.

Edith

At ninety, Edith still volunteered at the local animal shelter. However, one day at home she put an egg on to boil and then suddenly collapsed to the floor. Hours later, with the water boiled away, the egg exploded.

Eventually, Edith's grandson stopped by, found her, and called for an ambulance. At the hospital, tests revealed that she had suffered a major stroke, and that she had so much brain damage, recovery was unlikely. She was alert off and on, but she didn't stay awake long enough to take anything by mouth. She could not speak much more than a few words, but she nodded to questions appropriately.

Her advanced directives were readily available. She had named a healthcare proxy to make healthcare decisions in the event that she became incapable of doing so herself, and this person was quickly located and informed of Edith's status. Both in writing and through previous discussions with the proxy, Edith had left clear directions about just this type of circumstance. She did not want to have her life prolonged by artificial measures beyond IV hydration for short-term use.

During the next few days, healthcare staff provided her with IV fluids to see if she would have some return of neurologic function, and she also received some physical therapy. When there was no improvement, the staff explained the situation and choices to her healthcare proxy and to Edith. She was awake, seemed to understand, and they both agreed to pursue only comfort measures—interventions that are limited to the aim of promoting comfort and preventing suffering.

The IV ran its course. When it became dislodged, it was not replaced. During these final days, Edith took sips of water for pleasure, smiled, and watched the world around her. She seemed comfortable. Her family experienced some of the early stages of grief, but everyone understood that this was her wish. She sat up in a chair for several hours a day until she became too tired to do so, then stayed in bed until she died peacefully, surrounded by the ones she loved.

Healthcare decisions, especially related to long-term or custodial care, have potentially huge emotional and financial implications. Love, guilt, respect, entitlement, duty, and greed are all powerful forces. Combine this with sibling rivalry, family business, beloved and valuable homes, substance abuse, estrangements, and stepfamily dynamics, and there can be some stormy times. Having an overall goal that the family has agreed to will help when patients and their relatives are faced with a steady stream of health-related issues and decisions.

* * *

Elders who still live independently at home often have one primary wish—to remain there. The next two chapters look at ways to help them meet this goal for as long as they possibly can.

Chapter Two

Approaches to Care

While identifying goals for care may be fairly straightforward, it can be much more difficult for patients and their families to know how to achieve those goals. Complex medical problems often have several options for diagnosis and for treatment, and consequently more decisions may need to be made. In fact, as a medical situation evolves, even the simplest diagnosis can have a number of treatment options. This is why caregivers and healthcare providers need a suitable and individualized approach to making a plan for care. We will explore the most common approaches throughout this chapter and consider the pros and cons of each.

As I've emphasized so far, the more informed and directed patients and their caregivers are, the better the chances for a good outcome. However, this statement raises an essential question: *What is a good outcome?* Consider this question in respect to those of very advanced age and/or generalized frailty. Ultimately, death is the guaranteed outcome. However, the variables of choice can in a large degree help to determine the circumstances of death. In other words, by making compassionate, educated decisions, families and caregivers can help ensure that the ancient one's final experiences are mainly positive.

Each individual's preferred end-of-life scenario involves issues such as X, Y, Z. Some people may have contemplated these choices throughout their lives. Other people may never have considered their options or felt they had the luxury to make them. In any case, as life continues, decisions will need to be made. Consequently, the questions become, *By whom?* and *For whose benefit?*

The first question, *by whom?* has many possible answers—and many possible challenges. Family members may be in charge, due to patient incapacitation. At times, they may be unhappy with the direction the care is taking, or they may disagree with each other about the appropriate approach. There may be confusion about the overall plan of care. Family members can get frustrated and demanding if they don't feel that the providers are answering their questions effectively. Insecurity can also result in poor communication, which promotes even more insecurity and less comfort for the patients and loved ones.

The question of *by whom?* also overlaps with the question of *for whose benefit?* Without clarity in goals and approaches, there is the potential for patients to receive more, less, or different care than they desire. Sometimes in these situations, particularly when there is family discord, even the providers may act defensive or withdraw from discussions. However, this type of situation indicates the need for *more* discussion, not less. Family–team meetings are particularly useful in these situations, with all the involved parties—including the healthcare providers—gathering to make decisions together.

On its own, the question of *for whose benefit?* can also seem complicated. Much of healthcare focuses on the future, with early disease identification and treatment, long-term risk reduction, and complication prevention. However, the ancient ones may have a different perspective. Their future may not be as important to them as their present. Their medical status may limit the testing or treatment options that are available, or the elders themselves may simply refuse medical evaluation or treatment because they are indifferent to the possible outcome or they wish to avoid the degree of difficulty involved in the diagnostic process. Even if age is not a limiting factor, the reality is that frailty, regardless of age, can very much be a limiting factor in many courses of treatment.

To determine the best approach, patients and their caregivers need to review all the factors and related decisions. Keeping the goal in mind at all times will simplify the decision-making process and will result in the creation of a thoughtful plan of care rather than a series of disconnected interventions.

Lucy's Story

Before we go any further, let's take a look at Lucy's story. It highlights several common approaches both to the options for the diagnostic phase of evaluating the problem and to the options for the corresponding treatment.

Lucy

Lucy was a vibrant, ninety-five-year-old woman living fairly independently in the house she had been born in, complete with ocean view. She still went out, climbed stairs, smoked, sang sea shanties, and enjoyed rum at cocktail hour. As a woman of means, she had staff to provide daily assistance, take her on errands, and drive her to the doctor. Her family was not especially involved in her health care, but they really did not need to be.

One evening Lucy fell and broke her hip. She had surgery to repair the fracture and then was admitted to a facility for rehab. Initially, she was pleasant, spunky, and doing well. In the hospital she had been temporarily confused, but that had cleared up even before she arrived at rehab. Her goal, which was easy to identify, was to return to her baseline functional status and return home.

During her rehab, however, Lucy developed a mild pneumonia and a urinary tract infection, followed by lethargy and confusion. The doctors ordered oral antibiotics, and her physical therapy continued at a slower pace. Then she fell and bumped her head. At that point, she said she was "too tired" and uninterested in therapy, preferring to stay in bed. Naturally, her family became very concerned.

A family–team meeting was set up to discuss her status and to determine if the team needed to revise her original goal. Two of her children were serving as her healthcare proxies; the other two joined to share their ideas. As the following list shows, each of these family members favored a different approach to the possible steps for Lucy's care.

- The oldest, a scientist, advocated aggressive diagnostics and treatments. He focused on the possibility that much of this concerned the bump to the head. Did she need a CT scan to evaluate for a brain bleed? Was her decline a result of the head injury? Was she a candidate for neurosurgery, however minor? Did providers need any more information about her condition to plan a course of treatment? He adopted the "find it, fix it" approach, which promotes testing to identify a problem and then taking all possible steps to treat it. For example, he advocated getting a CT scan to rule in or rule out the worst case scenario (a brain problem such as a bleed, which could be treated with surgery); maintaining adequate fluids with IVs if needed; and inserting a feeding tube if eating was insufficient. Using this approach, he insisted that if the tests indicated a brain bleed, then surgery would be performed. Alternately, if the tests identified any infections, then those would be treated with antibiotics either by mouth or IV. If his siblings also adopted this approach, then they would try at all costs to keep Lucy's boat afloat. (Note that this could easily have evolved into a "never say die" approach, in which all possible steps are taken whether they are advisable or not.)

- One daughter seemed to think that the doctors should make the decision. She simply wanted to be told what to do—a "father knows best" approach.
- The middle daughter adopted a "life is good" approach to diagnosis and a "care and comfort" approach to treatment. She felt that the only interventions used should be ones that reduced Lucy's suffering. She was reluctant to try to get her mother to do anything she didn't want to do. Following this approach, if Lucy was tired, then she should be left in bed. If Lucy didn't want to do her exercises, that was fine. If her siblings adopted these approaches, there wouldn't be a CT scan.
- The third daughter wanted all the information available to make decisions. This "know the unknown" approach involves (1) testing to obtain the diagnosis; (2) scheduling further meetings to consider possible treatments and alternatives; and then (3) limiting some of the options.

In Lucy's case, what appears to be the best approach? A diagnosis can minimize uncertainty of cause, but improved outcome remains no sure thing. The diagnostic work-up itself may have unintended consequences—from the constipation from the dyes used in imaging studies, to the exhausting discomfort from the long ambulance or wheelchair ride to learn about a surgery no one wants or advises. The circumstance is more perilous if sedation is required for compliance to complete diagnostic testing.

> Working together, the family concluded that at ninety-five, Lucy had lived a full, wonderful life. Not only was she showing signs of giving up, but she appeared to be okay with that decision.
>
> After speaking with the medical team, the family also recognized the possibility that Lucy might not even have a brain injury or a treatable condition. It was possible that she was simply very tired and that even with no more than "comfort measures," Lucy might stabilize. The siblings agreed that providers would encourage fluids and food (ice cream three times a day if she desired), oral medications, and gentle exercises as tolerated. Providers would follow Lucy's lead, plan her day accordingly, treat her symptoms as they presented themselves, and wait to see what happened next.

As Lucy's family adopted this care-and-comfort approach, they braced for her death. However, Lucy's situation stabilized, and with hospice care she was able to return to her ocean-view home. Her new plan included rest, plenty of music, a lot of sweets, and a weak evening cocktail. Two years later, hospice long gone, she was still alive, although at ninety-seven, she finally quit smoking.

Hospice

The word *hospice* refers to a philosophy of care, as well as a specific organization of care providers.

As a philosophical framework, *hospice* describes care with a primary function of providing supportive end-of-life ministrations for individuals and their families. Medical care is focused on treating symptoms, maintaining dignity, and preventing suffering. It is an interdisciplinary approach and helps support the patient, as well as all those affected by the difficult dying process.

As an organization, hospice is usually a covered insurance benefit for those who meet the criteria. This includes assistance from a specialized team of doctors, nurses, nurses' aides, social workers, and chaplains. Sometimes the hospice team also includes massage and music therapists, trained dogs, and child development specialists.

The hospice team will augment the ancient one's established medical team, and its members can take on a leadership role in the medical management of these patients. Hospice care, which may or may not occur in the patient's home, is episodic, meaning that hospice workers make visits to perform assessments, make recommendations, or provide a specific service, such as bathing or wound care. It does not provide twenty-four hour care. Other arrangements need to be made for the "around-the-clock" care and medication administration, which can be performed in the home by hospice-supervised and supported family members, friends, or paid nursing staff.

Hospice care can also be provided in the hospital or freestanding hospice houses. These settings are usually reserved for management of difficult symptoms, or with a life expectancy measured in days. Hospice care also occurs in nursing homes, either with a long-term patient who has declined or with a person in the community whose care can no longer be managed at home. Again, the hospice care is an addition to the routine care provided by regular staff.

The recognition of who is "ready" for hospice is not always an easy task. The specific criteria for hospice changes, but in general a life expectancy of six months or less is usually needed for the patient to qualify. Because that timeline is unpredictable, other guidelines may be used, such as the presence of a terminal or end-stage illness, informed refusal of a life-sustaining treatment, or advanced dementia with weight loss. It is not uncommon for a person to meet criteria for hospice but then improve, gain weight and strength over time, and no longer qualify for hospice care. At that point the person transitions back to routine care as appropriate. This was the case with Lucy.

The Most Common Approaches

The following section describes the most common approaches to treating the ancient ones, along with some of the pros and cons of each (Figure 3-1). I have identified and grouped these approaches (or patterns of behavior) based on years of observing patients and their advocates make their way through the healthcare maze.

Approach	Key Features	Pros	Cons
Life Is Good	Accepts changes of all kinds. Expects changes to occur.	Adjusts goals and approaches as circumstances change.	None.
Find It, Fix It	Advocates for evaluation of all symptoms. Screens for asymptomatic problems. Expects and accepts no limits on treatment options.	Considers standard of care regardless of advanced age or frailty. Avoids "failure to diagnose."	Patient may receive duplicate, unnecessary, or futile care. Patient may suffer pain, indignity, or other unpleasant consequences of care.
Never Say Die	Strives for longevity at any cost.	Exhausts all options of care.	Patient's suffering is not a limiting factor to ongoing treatment. Patient may receive futile care.
Know the Unknown	Wants an explanation or clear diagnosis for problems.	Obtains a diagnosis. Provides family with patient's medical history.	Doesn't affect or alter the treatment plan. May suffer adverse effects from testing.
Father Knows Best	Follows medical advice without question.	Easy patient or caregiver for providers to deal with. Compliant and satisfied with any decision.	May be directed against the patient's true wishes.
Live Free or Die	Reluctantly makes compromises.	Maintains sense of control.	May make dangerous or unwise decisions.
Don't Ask, Don't Tell	Does not seek healthcare nor volunteer information.	Privacy is maintained.	May obscure a diagnosis, delay treatment.
Care and Comfort	Immediate quality of life is focus. Does not want much diagnostic evaluation.	Suffering or discomfort is minimized.	May forgo treatment for a treatable condition.

Note that many of these approaches occur sequentially or concurrently. Medical situations are often complex, and changes may happen quickly. Plans need to be made for the situations that patients and caregivers want to have happen (Plan A) but also for those that are actually happening (Plan B).

Patients, caregivers, and healthcare providers who learn to recognize the different features of the range of common approaches can use this knowledge as a reference point to help make decisions and to provide a context for addressing the obstacles to goal achievement. As you read the examples in the pages that follow, you will note again that the approaches can—and often do—overlap. However, for instructional purposes, each story will focus on one key aspect of the different approaches.

LIFE IS GOOD

A major part of the "life is good" approach involves the patient's and family's appreciation for the ancient one's current stage in life.

Mrs. Elliot

At ninety-three, Mrs. Elliot, independent and thriving, was still living what appeared to be a charmed life. Healthy, wealthy, and wise, she was very kind and was loved by many. Then doctors found a mass in her abdomen during a routine checkup. Using noninvasive imaging studies (ultrasound and CT scan), doctors determined the mass was cancer.

Mrs. Elliot was faced with the decision of how to proceed. Within her there was a known cancer. It was causing her no trouble or symptoms, but it might speed up and kill her. Should she submit herself to a surgery that would clearly decrease her day-to-day quality of life for several months? Major surgery is no picnic at any age, but it's an enormous undertaking at ninety-three. After lengthy discussion and consultations with family and her primary care physician, she decided to follow a "life is good" approach: In the absence of symptoms, she would forego surgery and enjoy life as always.

People like Mrs. Elliot are such a joy to know. They live every minute of their lives, making constant accommodations for life's ever-changing drama. Bad things happen; they deal with them and then they just move on. Little things remain little things, and their awareness focuses on life's bounty rather than on its scarcity. When they are in the hospital, they enjoy the nurses and the housekeeping staff. Medically they stay interested in prevention practices, eating prudently to stay healthy, being flexible, and changing the menu to keep up with the times. Taking yoga for balance sounds like fun, and they sign up for a class. They keep their brains active with bridge, classes, crossword puzzles, and discussion groups. They ask questions and care about others. They think carefully about how decisions to prolong a poor quality of life may impact others, and they remain realistic when faced with a poor prognosis. Their attitude runs along the lines of "I've lived my life and it has been good; it is okay to die, and I am at peace."

> As time progressed, Mrs. Elliot combined the "life is good" approach with the "name the trouble" approach. She continued to have her doctors monitor the behavior of her cancer through regular scans and blood work. When she developed some abdominal pain, the corresponding change in the tests indicated disease progression.
>
> Because Mrs. Elliot's main goal was to continue to enjoy her life as fully as possible ("life is good"), she eventually decided to have the surgery to buy her time and slow the cancer's progression. Using her resources and connections she was able to hire good help at home and slowly recovered. Though weakened and much frailer, she retained her spark. Two months post-op, she was able to resume many of her usual activities, and she enjoyed relatively good health once again for more than a year. At that point, when the abdominal pain returned, she accepted the situation and switched her goal to a "care and comfort" approach. She started pain medication and received hospice care until she peacefully died at home.

FIND IT, FIX IT

The "find it, fix it" approach represents the standard path medical care follows. It focuses on early identification of diseases followed by prompt treatment, with the goal of curing the disease, limiting disease progression, or preventing complications. It is also the approach taken with the evaluation of every problem or symptom.

With the "find it, fix it" approach toward healthcare, there are few, if any, limits on treatment options. (Issues of insurance limitations are not included in this discussion.) No test or diagnostic procedure is deferred due to difficulty or inconvenience. Medical treatment is aimed at correcting or managing the defect. There is the assumption that good or improved health happens with the correct chemistry, the right numbers, and the absence of pathology. This is exactly the right approach for patients to take when they need it. However, the key is to know when they need it.

Peter

Peter was a robust, vibrant man in his early eighties. He had survived four hip replacements, various hernia repairs, vascular surgeries, cardiac bypass surgery, and a nasty cancer, proudly displaying surgical scars from the top of his chest to his ankle. A kind, lighthearted fighter, he was as tough as they come. Whatever health problem he encountered, he overcame. His approach was clearly "find it, fix it."

A month-long hospitalization, which was related to the cancer, might have ended with hospice care, but not for Peter. He went home to live, not to die. Peter had sported a physique like a Greek God as a younger man, so he was now miffed to be given two-pound weights to rebuild his body, but he did it slowly, all day, every day.

Gradually he gained weight and strength and was able to resume the outdoor work that he loved, gardening and even using the chainsaw. However, after a period of time, he became very sick and was brought back to a big city hospital to have the most aggressive treatment available. Progressive cancer left him in pain, nauseated, and unable to eat or drink. He was misery personified. His pain was severe and the narcotics worsened his bowel problem and made him confused. The only hope for even a little more time was surgery to relieve the bowel obstruction. However, the odds were not in his favor. There was only a 50–50 chance of surviving the operation, and it was not going to be a long-term fix.

At this point, many people would have chosen a different approach, such as a "care and comfort" approach. However, Peter's approach to his life was echoed in his approach to his death. Surviving serious illnesses in the past had prepared him for further survival. It seemed like it almost didn't occur to him that there would be a time he would not live to see another day. He was full of a sense of curiosity and was willing to keep at the experiment until it was successful or just couldn't go on.

Loving life, he elected to proceed with the surgery. At this point, the "find it, fix it" approach seemed to be losing ground, and it started to look like a "never say die" approach was moving in. He survived the surgery, but his symptoms did not improve, and to make matters worse, he had a lot of post-op pain to endure.

Peter had a very scientific, experimental approach to life, jury-rigging many a gizmo in his time when others would have given up. It made sense to him that the doctors should take the same approach with him. The doctors worked hard to keep him going when all his organs seemed to be failing. This is the type of care patients receive at a major medical center. It's the hospital's job.

During Peter's final hours, a "do not resuscitate" order was instituted just in time. He died hooked up to all kinds of monitors, but not life support.

One of the drawbacks to the "find it, fix it" approach is that many problems exist that are not easy to identify. Consequently, at any point along the way, patients and their providers may consult with multiple specialists in the particular area of concern for either the diagnosis or the treatment plan. This may involve the patient being transferred to a major medical center for either ongoing hospital treatment or outpatient care. A complicated patient may end up with quite an assortment of specialists. It would not be surprising to have duplication of testing as each specialist may not have knowledge of, or access to, previous diagnostic studies. In these situations it is very important to have a primary care physician (PCP) kept up to date on all specialist visits to maintain a complete picture of what is going on.

With this approach, it is not uncommon for the medically complex ancient ones to feel that their life revolves around the ongoing medical monitoring. In a sense, it sometimes seems that healthcare providers are maintaining the life of complicated elderly patients in order to continue to monitor and treat their conditions, leaving the ancient ones with precious little time to enjoy the life that is being preserved. With "find it, fix it" models, there is a "leave no stone unturned" approach when seeking an answer or a diagnosis, and a "what have I got to lose" attitude when determining treatments.

All of this testing may also result in the identification of problems unrelated to the symptom being evaluated. For example, an x-ray taken to look for a broken bone after a fall may show something in the belly or lungs that looks like a cancer. Sometimes these incidental findings are beneficial, but sometimes they simply take patients on a very prolonged and uncomfortable detour as providers work up one abnormal finding after another.

Another shortcoming of the "find it, fix it" approach is that when nothing is found, there is nothing apparent to fix. The symptoms persist and yet, since doctors can't find an explanation, the course of action remains unclear. The new goal may be to identify treatment plans for the relief of symptoms and how to function in the presence of these symptoms. The "progression of chronic conditions" ends up being used as an explanation for a wide range of symptoms, especially when a work-up yields little more than which conditions have been ruled out.

NEVER SAY DIE

"Never say die" describes an approach in which extraordinary measures are taken after a problem is identified but not able to be solved. It involves the ongoing treatment of a person who almost certainly won't get better but goes to great lengths to "beat the odds."

Patricia

Patricia, in her late seventies, lost her ability to care for herself—a task she had never embraced fully in the first place. Morbidly obese, anxious, and depressed, she had poorly controlled diabetes, high blood pressure, and bad arthritis in her hips and knees, which had kept her homebound for years. She had terrible troubles with swelling, infection, and sores in her legs as she spent most of her day sitting in a chair with legs down. She was a regular with the visiting nurses, and she had an occasional hospitalization.

After one admission, she went into rehab again, but this time she wasn't able or willing to participate with therapy. Consequently, she was unable to get out of her chair or perform her most basic activities of daily living (ADLs). It became clear that she could not return to living home alone. Instead she stayed at the rehab center for long-term custodial care, and she took to her bed. Surrounded by stuffed animals, she happily enjoyed her meals, which were placed on the bedside tray. Ironically, her legs, which had caused so much trouble with swelling, infection, and sores when she lived at home, were much improved once she "took to her bed" because they were elevated.

Patricia still had frequent infections: skin, respiratory, and urinary tract. With multiple antibiotic allergies and the development of resistant germs, her infections became more serious and more difficult to treat. She suffered two heart attacks and a small stroke, and she was staying sicker longer, lengthening her periodic hospital stays. Upon her return to rehab, her goals were for bed mobility only, as she was still unable or unwilling to get out of bed. In fact, it took her great effort to regain the strength to reposition herself in bed.

To those who witnessed Patricia's experiences, this seemed like a poor quality of life, particularly as she was confined to bed in a nursing home. Still, she never wanted to give up on medical treatment. She took the "never say die" approach. When her kidneys failed and the only option for survival was dialysis, she got hooked up. Three times per week she went via ambulance to dialysis, forty-five minutes away, to be plugged in for five hours. She suffered from motion sickness and needed medication or else she would vomit during the trip. As the years went by, the dialysis access sites in her body deteriorated and she needed multiple procedures to maintain the capability for ongoing treatment. In spite of the chronic pain and nausea, shortness of breath, and dizziness, she chose to continue this life by sustaining treatment as long as possible.

The "never say die" approach does not consider death to be an acceptable option due to the perception of the patient, the family, or seemingly, the providers. This is taking the "find it, fix it" approach to extremes. The problem has been found but there may be no remedy. Medical interventions are undertaken to prolong life at any cost. Quality of life or comfort is not the goal; staying alive is.

This approach is often selected in response to a sudden change of status that is due to a specific event, such as stroke or trauma. In other cases, it is followed throughout a slow decline from progressive disease, such as heart and lung disease or cancer.

Our health care system offers patients opportunities to continue with life-sustaining treatments and strenuous efforts for therapy even when there is progressive and severe disease combined with physical suffering. Along the same lines, patients or their health care proxies who refuse to accept that death is inevitable may decide to withhold or forego comfort measures such as pain medication in order to avoid side effects such as sleepiness or confusion.

For families, caregivers, and providers, there is always the balance of trying to maintain hope for the patients while—at the same time—trying to "keep it real." False or hollow reassurance will benefit no one. If the damage is widespread or the suffering is severe, then these issues may outweigh the benefit from continuing life-sustaining treatment.

Needless to say, the "never say die" approach can create a lot of turmoil for providers and family members who disagree with it. Even when information and guidance is available, there is no requirement for patients and their health proxies to accept it.

When I am working with a patient who I believe is needlessly suffering, I invite the healthcare agent to witness the daily events. This alone can be very persuasive. If it is not, and no changes in the plan are made, then I ensure that there is ongoing communication about status changes in either direction—improvements or failings—in the hope that informed decisions can start to be made in the near future.

There are several reasons why the "never say die" approach continues to be offered and practiced in modern medicine. First, there are conflicting values in medical care between the sworn "do no harm" and cover your anatomy ("CYA"). This is done in part to avoid the accusation of "failure to treat." Ordering tests and treatments can seem proper, easier, and oftentimes less time-consuming than the long discussion often needed as these situations develop. Yet responsible healthcare providers should feel obligated to talk with patients and their representatives when harm seems to outweigh benefit.

Religious beliefs may also have a large impact in these issues, and clergy may help facilitate these conversations. Different faiths will have different points of view about what is considered ordinary versus extraordinary care, the meaning of suffering, and quality-of-life issues. Hospital-based ethics committees exist to allow for the representation of all sides of a situation, while keeping the focus on the patient at all times. In extreme cases when there is no consensus, the courts have to decide these difficult issues.

Fear of death, feelings of guilt, and a strong sense of potential betrayal are also common reasons that patients and their caregivers choose to pursue medical interventions at all costs. Of course, these feelings are completely understandable; no one wants to lose a loved one, and no one wants to feel like it is his or her fault. Decision makers may feel as if they are betraying the patient by not fighting to the very last moment or by passively allowing the loved one to die. Patients and caregivers alike may fear the suffering they expect to occur with the dying process.

In these cases, death education may help to allay these concerns and fears. For example, it's important for patients, families, and health proxies to understand that just because the eventuality of death is accepted and routine care is discontinued, this does not mean that the medical personnel are "doing nothing." I frequently find myself explaining that the alternative approach of comfort measures at the end of life *is* "doing something." In fact, end-of-life care, which is discussed in Chapter 11, is a very different approach from doing nothing. There is no reason for the perpetuation of suffering to become "routine."

Are there times when a patient turns an unexpected corner and makes some degree of recovery following the "never say die" approach? Yes, I've certainly seen that happen. However, because it tends to be the exception versus the rule, I encourage patients and their caregivers to carefully weigh all of the options, goals, and changes in condition before sticking resolutely to *any* plan that may simply prolong suffering.

KNOW THE UNKNOWN

"Know the Unknown" is an approach that involves seeking all available information about the problem. This is the first half of the "find it, fix it" approach. There is a careful consideration of current status and overall prognosis with just enough diagnostic testing to help the decision-making process. This is often sensible and can provide peace of mind for family members when thinking and rethinking about the medical details. They may be reassured by knowing, for sure, that there was no useful or reasonable treatment available for their loved one. There is also the issue of family medical history; people often want to know who died of what, and how that affects the surviving family members. Rosa's story offers one example.

Rosa

Rosa, who appeared to suffer from dementia, was a ninety-five-year-old Italian-speaking, deaf, arthritic woman with low vision. She was loved dearly by her numerous children, who visited for hours every day. They seemed to be able to communicate with her, sorting out her ramblings from the requests for Italian ice.

When she began to decline, they were mystified, "How can it be?" they asked. Yet such a global decline is not unusual. Progressive dementia with weight loss, swallowing problems, an occasional respiratory tract infection, and a GI bleed is not uncommon. First, the acute problems clear up readily and then, as time progresses, less readily.

In Rosa's case, the chronic problems, which seemed mostly related to the dementia and arthritis of hips and knees, progressed. She required more and more assistance as her walking and self-grooming abilities got worse.

Eventually, when Rosa developed asymptomatic rectal bleeding, the family chose to pursue the cause ("know the unknown"), even though she was unable to comprehend the problem or the purpose and procedures of the recommended tests. She had multiple physical exams of the area, with increasing anxiety, and then a colonoscopy, which involves scopes inserted through the rectum into the colon. Like many diagnostic tests, a colonoscopy requires bowel prep, which requires the consumption of large amounts of laxatives on a schedule in order to empty all stools from the body; this is often quite a large amount. With many trips to the bathroom it is a long and exhausting process to say the least.

For Rosa, side effects from the sedating medication, which was required for the most unpleasant parts, resulted in persistent lethargy and restless agitation, and lasted for almost a week after the procedure. The results indicated colon cancer. The family then decided to forego further diagnostic testing to determine the cell type and presence and/or extent of spread. They also decided to decline possible treatments (surgical or chemotherapy) and moved on to a "care and comfort" approach.

Rosa's story illustrates a common problem: A frail elder presents with a group of symptoms that are likely to be caused by cancer. With the "know the unknown" approach, the patient and family may decide not to pursue treatment, but they still want a formal diagnosis, which may provide them with a degree of clarity as far as prognosis and expected course of the disease.

Still, as Rosa's story shows, this diagnosis can come at a high price, particularly when possible treatment is removed from the equation. More specific information may not be useful, since the testing itself has a degree of risk and will not change the plan of treatment or expected outcome. Rosa was put through an ordeal that was stressful both mentally and physically in order to name the problem, even though in the end the family decided not to pursue treatment for the diagnosed ailment.

In some cases, the medical team may advise against the "know the unknown" approach. At times, there is no benefit from knowing the precise diagnosis because none of the possibilities have positive outcomes. As an example, let's look at Billy's story.

Billy

Billy, a ninety-four-year-old man who was staying in a rehabilitation facility after a stroke, was taken to the emergency room with symptoms of nausea, vomiting, abdominal pain, and distention. An abdominal cat scan (CT) revealed a large mass located near his pancreas. From the healthcare providers' standpoint, it was very clear that this was one of several very bad possibilities. The physicians did not feel it would be useful to make a firm diagnosis, as nothing about it seemed fixable.

Billy suffered from mild dementia and did not have the mental capability to make medical decisions. The "care and comfort" option was presented to the family with the suggestion for hospice care, focusing on the expected development of distressing symptoms. Yet Billy, in spite of it all, had started feeling better. The bowel obstruction resolved, and his other issues, which included a urinary tract infection and anemia, were treated successfully. He returned to the nursing home back at his baseline condition (stroke patient with dementia) oblivious to the fact of the new—presumed terminal—diagnosis.

However, while Billy seemed to be back on track, his nephew was experiencing significantly more distress regarding the lack of a specific diagnosis. Billy's nephew wanted no stone left unturned about diagnosis and treatment options. He wanted a second opinion and stated that he was not ready for the care-and-comfort plan. He wanted Billy to undergo a biopsy to provide an exact tissue diagnosis, and he wanted to hear the options of how this could be obtained and the condition ultimately treated.

These ideas put Billy's nephew at odds with some of the healthcare providers. Ultimately, after an oncology conference with Billy's primary care doctor and cancer specialists, who unanimously agreed that a biopsy would be pro-hibitively difficult and provide no useful information for the care of the patient, the nephew agreed to hospice care. Doctors assured him that if he continued to have lingering concerns about family medical history, an autopsy could be performed after Billy's death. Currently, Billy is at the nursing home enjoying the time he has left, unaware of the dramas undertaken on his behalf.

FATHER KNOWS BEST

The "Father knows best" approach involves the patient's and/or family members' demonstra-tion of the utmost trust for the doctor or other provider and the medical system in general. This is a passive—and often optimistic—approach. The patients get their check-ups because they are supposed to. They rarely look up information in books, magazines, or on the Internet; nor do they ask for a second opinion. Details are not important. They are compliant patients, satisfied and satisfying. They won't ask many questions or inquire about options. They may not even care to know if there are options. In the delegation of these choices, there is also the freedom of responsibility and accountability about the consequences of these actions.

People who adopt this approach feel that "Decisions are best made by those professionals who know best." They often seem confused about why their own "lay" opinions might be sought. These patients may not have a clear understanding of their conditions or medications, including names and doses; they may not even want to understand. Intelligence or educa-tion does not seem to be a factor in this approach. It always surprises me to see intelligent, educated people refer to their meds by color, size, and shape rather than by name, dose, or function. The main difficulty with the "Father knows best" approach occurs when patients or their families need to make a decision, particularly a major treatment decision, because they feel (and are) unprepared to do so.

I think this trait represents either great trust in the medical establishment or obliviousness to the reality that patients may one day find themselves in a situation where they need to be knowledgeable enough about their own circumstances to provide a medical history, as in an unanticipated medical encounter. (Conversely, intrinsically suspicious people will know every nuance of med changes; they are constantly aware, and reminding me, that another medical calamity is around the corner.)

People who rely on the "Father knows best" approach often deal with healthcare decisions by asking the provider, "What would you do if this were your [brother, mother, grandparent]?" This seems to be another way of asking, "What should I do?"

Another type of "Father knows best" approach is the devout spiritual belief that God knows and cares about every person's health status. It can be hard to pin down patients' wishes and goals when they are quite sure that God is taking care of all these details. This approach can take several different directions. For instance, some people believe that CPR and other aggressive medical care is God's will; others believe it is trying to get in the way of God's will.

Simon

"Ninety-five is much older than ninety," Simon told visitors at his assisted living facility. He was a gifted and prolific artist, the quintessential gentleman who had led a structured, sensible life. Heart trouble in his forties convinced him of the importance of prudent habits. For more than fifty years his healthy habits included a routine of calisthenics in the early morning, focused work, brisk walks, and, in the summer, frequent swims. Eating habits were very structured, and he ate his three meals at the same time daily, with all of the advised low-fat meats and generous portions of fruit and vegetables. He drank skim milk and a quart of water daily. To help him sleep, he recited poetry he had memorized as a child. When his eyes began to fail in his early nineties, he gave up his beloved art, but he simply turned this into an opportunity to reflect upon his long and productive life, and he concentrated on writing his memoirs.

Although generally in good health, he had several medical conditions, which were well controlled. He was a very compliant patient. Visits to the doctor were regularly scheduled, pleasurable excursions and a source of comfort and reassurance. Medicines to be taken on an empty stomach were taken on an empty stomach. When advised to put his feet up for twenty minutes, he would set the timer. He had a "Father knows best" approach to his healthcare, and "doctor's orders" were the supreme rule. In fact, he would often seek approval or permission to use this authority to cancel meetings and otherwise modify his schedule. "Don't you think it would be too tiring for me?" or "Aren't visits best kept under twenty minutes?" he would hopefully ask.

As time passed, Simon recognized his own physical and intellectual decline, however slight they seemed to others. By ninety-seven, he was frail but as charming as ever. That year, in early winter, he fell and broke his wrist. He had discomfort and needed help with the activities of daily living. He was told he needed a caregiver and he readily agreed. He tolerated—even enjoyed—this attention, but only as a novel experience, not anything he wanted to become a habit.

Simon's family joined him for a quiet and pleasant holiday. Shortly after, they noticed that he seemed to be losing his interest in eating his food. He would say, "Oh it smells wonderful and looks better," but he had no inclination to eat it.

At that point, Simon began asking the purpose of each med he took and the expected outcome of discontinuing it. Eventually he asked if it was okay to simply stop taking them. His providers assured him that it was his choice to take or not take his meds, and his family agreed that his choices would be honored.

His family made him his favorite soup, and the savory aroma filled his home. The medical team warned him that he should not expect a sudden effect from stopping the meds, but they were wrong. Within two days he died peacefully, comfortably at home in his own bed, family at his side, and a slight smile on his face.

Simon's quick death was surprising to me at the time, but later, as I reflected upon it, I saw how his "Father knows best" approach affected his death. His faith in the absolute correctness of his medical care was probably more life-sustaining than the medications themselves. The combination of stopping his meds and the "permission" to do so allowed him to peacefully slip away.

When we consider the ramifications of the "Father knows best" approach, we see that on the one hand, there are not a lot of choices, because the patient effortlessly accepts the advised care. On the other hand, there are choices when it comes to picking the healthcare provider that the patient is going to rely on. It is especially important for patients with this attitude to have a compatible healthcare provider. Frail elders need a primary care provider to direct them toward the care that is appropriate for them based on their individual wants and needs.

LIVE FREE OR DIE

The "live free or die" (or "homeward bound") approach follows the belief that the ultimate goal in life is independence or self-determination. People who feel this way go to doctors and tell them what they want and what they are willing to do. They may refuse medications because it cramps their style, their pocketbook, or their idea of themselves. There is rigidity in this way of thinking that makes compromises undesirable and infrequent.

This value system can set up seemingly unnecessary obstacles to even simple suggestions. People with this approach may be so set in their ways that they resist modification of their diets, habits, or patterns of activity. Their attitude is that life is to be lived on their own terms or it's not worth living. The use of cigarettes and excessive alcohol are obvious examples of this approach; people decide that these pleasures are worth the risk, and they avoid seeking medical advice because they deem it to be predictable and unappealing. Their typical response is, "The doctor will just tell me to quit and I'm not going to."

A common thought with this approach is, "I'd rather die than live with _____." Here we can fill in the blank with *dementia, blindness, paralysis,* or just about any medical situation, disability, or situational change. A common example is, "I'd rather die than live in a nursing home." This philosophy sets up big problems for those caregivers who are developing a plan for patients who have been declared unsafe and yet want to return home, particularly when the patients have been deemed "competent" to make decisions—including bad ones.

Ancient ones who take this approach tend to resist even the most commonsense, practical suggestions. For instance, maybe family members have identified areas in the home or self-care routines that increase the risk of injury, and they have made suggestions to change the décor or the procedure for the daily ablutions. Most of us would agree that it's worth it to accept such a small disruption in these routines in order to avoid the risk of a major problem. We would be willing to remove the scatter rugs because they aren't safe. We would rather start sitting down to put our socks on rather than fall, break a hip, and undergo hip surgery. Unfortunately, for people with a "live free or die" approach, the answer is quite often, "No."

Giving up driving may also become a major issue for these people. The ancient ones who take this approach will go to great extremes to maintain their driving privileges, often demonstrating a great capacity for rationalization to compensate for diminished driving skill. "I never go off the island. I stay off the highway. I avoid rush hour, dark, and rain." My favorite line comes from my own Aunt Mary: "I can see all the light-colored cars." Intervention may be an essential life saver in cases such as these. The personal choice of "live free or die" is one thing, but turning a car into a potential vehicle of mass destruction is another. Driving is discussed in Chapter 3.

When it comes to making medical choices, the "live free or die" approach is often temporary, and there seem to be two groups of patients: those who mean it and those who just say it. When there are suddenly choices to be made after a catastrophic event, such as a major stroke, an elder with this approach may consider what the future holds and simply stop eating. Yet another person faced with a similar situation may drop the "or die" like a hot potato and seek full treatment for all problems, shifting into another approach altogether.

The concept of suicide or physician-assisted suicide also comes up with the extreme manifestation of this approach. An utter intolerance for the physical realities of life, disease, or disability can prompt this "live free or die" final act. Legal and religious restrictions may also impact the activeness of the plan, from actual suicide to a slower death that occurs from the choice to opt out of food, fluids, or life-sustaining meds or treatments. These situations can at times be managed with the addition of hospice or other end-of-life specialty services.

Rachel's story, which follows, shows how complicated the "live free or die" situation can become, particularly when the ancient ones seem to switch back and forth between approaches and the families and medical providers either aren't really sure what the patients' wishes might be—or choose to override those wishes.

Rachel

Rachel was a woman in her mid-eighties who had lost her voice, first due to cancer of the throat and then, after a stroke, from aphasia, an impairment of verbal expression that caused her to struggle with comprehension and expression of thoughts much beyond the loss of voice. She also had lost the ability to read and write.

Although Rachel was able to live with her daughter for a short time, she began to suffer from social isolation, inactivity, and poor appetite. Falls also became both more frequent and more serious.

Within a year, Rachel was back at rehab for long-term care. It was clear that she was extremely unhappy about it, though really there was no alternative. Her depression was treated, as well as several medical events, including further stroke activity and worsening functional status over the next year or so.

With that in mind, her family and the medical team felt she had a fairly good comprehension of the world around her. She could nod, give thumbs up or thumbs down, and, with the depression managed successfully, was basically in a pretty good mood.

A recurring problem during this time was that Rachel hated to take pills and often refused them. Yet after several days of refusing diuretics (fluid retention pills) to keep her out of heart failure, she would invariably end up in acute heart failure. She would develop a panicky shortness of breath with a very tight chest, and she would consent in the end—before her end—to get the same medication she had been refusing all week long, in a quick-acting, injectable form. Symptoms would promptly resolve, and for a week or month she would be more compliant with her medications.

One day, Rachel clearly communicated that she wanted no more pills, including the antidepressants, and no more food. Basically, she indicated that she was creating a hunger strike (including medications) because she wanted OUT. She pointed to family photos to indicate she wanted to be with her deceased family members including her husband, parents, and son.

Her "hunger strike" went on quietly for a few days, then a week. She remained cheerful and even had an occasional milkshake with her daughter. But no joking, pleading, or crying got her to eat anything substantial. At that point, her physician stepped in and ordered a psychiatric evaluation, which purportedly determined that she was severely depressed and delusional (quite an assessment in a nonverbal woman). Remember that her problems with speaking were twofold: loss of voice (she had always refused to accept a speaking device), and the more problematic aphasia that disturbed her brain center of communication so that written expression was no better. She was committed to a locked psychiatric unit since her behavior was putting herself in mortal peril as she intentionally starved herself. She then came back to the rehabilitation facility on more meds—which she took—and she started eating.

Initially Rachel seemed happy again, and we were glad to see her improvement. However, as time progressed, she developed painful leg wounds from poor circulation. Basically, her legs were slowly dying. After Rachel and her daughter met with a surgeon, who offered options including amputation, which Rachel declined, she was switched to a "care and comfort" approach. As the circulation to her legs worsened, she required more pain medication. Ultimately, she died after much more anguish than the caregivers could prevent.

As family members, caregivers, and medical staff members, when do we honor an elder's "live free or die" approach, when do we insist on interventions, and when do we move on to a "care and comfort" approach? In the example above, honoring Rachel's first "hunger strike" might have spared her the entire miserable episode that occurred at the end of her life. While we cannot predict the future and cannot prevent all suffering, it is ironic that we often allow the choice for comfort measures only when somehow we feel that the ancient one has "suffered enough" before forfeiting treatment.

DON'T ASK, DON'T TELL

"Don't ask, don't tell" is a common approach among elders who are reluctant to interact with the healthcare system. They don't want to see a doctor or a nurse, let alone be seen by one. A caring friend or family member often brings these folks to the office or the emergency room. These ancient ones either think they are sick and may be beyond help, or they have no faith in the medical world and have no use for the experience. They are not happy to be there and are not forthcoming with information, thinking doctors are nosy. Even though they may be having significant symptoms, unless directly confronted, they may "forget" to mention major issues like chest pain or abnormal bleeding. Their lack of medical insight may cause them to fail to recognize an important symptom.

People who adopt this approach may also believe that it helps them avoid unwanted medical information. For instance, they might say, "If you never go to the doctor, it is unlikely that you will ever be told you have diabetes or cancer." People with this line of thinking often live in fear of diseases such as lung cancer, but they may continue to smoke and won't take advantage of screening tests to try to find diseases in early stages.

Healthcare providers are taught to inquire about a variety of symptoms through a process called "review of systems." However, people with the "don't ask, don't tell" approach are likely to slip through the cracks, particularly when healthcare providers do not conduct the review due to a lack of time, a lack of a common language, or just an oversight. This also occurs when patients do not provide information because they are confused, forgetful, fearful, mistrustful, or embarrassed. Issues such as substance use/abuse, domestic violence, sexuality, and bathroom habits are often overlooked topics in all age groups, and they are even less likely to be discussed among the elderly. Cultural differences between the patient and care providers can also have an impact in obtaining pertinent information.

It is often helpful for medical staff members to get supporting information from family members and direct care providers. However, it is important to recognize that this healthcare approach of "don't ask, don't tell" is also common with some caregivers—such as the spouses of sick patients—in terms of hiding their *own* symptoms. These caregivers frequently ignore or minimize their own symptoms because they fear that a diagnosed illness may result in the diminishment of their role or capacity to perform needed tasks. They feel that there's no time for them to be sick, so they discount this possibility. They may also downplay their loved one's illness because they blame themselves or fear the separation that could occur if the loved one needs to be hospitalized for treatment.

Another aspect to the "don't tell" approach involves caregivers who choose not to tell the patient the diagnosis. This can occur at the request of family members, who for some reason feel that the patient "can't handle it." In these situations, everyone except the patient knows that the patient has cancer, for example, and is going to die.

Is this ever an acceptable choice to make? I am never in favor of withholding a diagnosis from a mentally capable patient. However, it's possible that some patients with cognitive impairment don't want or need to know a lot of details about exactly how bad it is. For instance, if an intervention such as surgery has been ruled out and no major treatment is planned, is it important for patients to get more information about the specifics of how bad it is? Perhaps not. In these situations, healthcare staff can provide accurate information in pieces according to how much impact it has on whatever treatment *is* occurring.

In some situations, the patients actually seem to manage to forget that they have been given a poor prognosis. After one or two times of reminding them, the medical team and their caregivers may realize it isn't useful to repeat the information.

Pete

Pete was a skinny eighty-eight-year-old married man. He had been healthy for most of his life, with his biggest problems centering around his struggles with both anxiety and depression. Over the years he took many different medicines for this.

Pete was admitted to the hospital after multiple bouts of pneumonia. The latest episode was one of several in succession that ultimately left him too weak to walk, so he needed rehab. He knew he was "scrawny" but said he usually "got along okay."

Pete progressed well in therapy, but then the staff noted that he made a funny sound while speaking, and they noticed vomiting on many occasions after meals. The staff discovered that he had made it through numerous doctors' appointments and two hospitalizations without anyone identifying this ailment, which had been going on for years with increasing frequency and intensity.

Pete had never shared this information with healthcare providers because he viewed the situation as a quirk more than a problem. He and his wife seemed to think it too distasteful or even insignificant to discuss. As well, "medical business" made him nervous, and all of his symptoms worsened when he was nervous.

When the medical staff tried to discuss the situation with Pete, he did not volunteer many specifics. He and his wife had grown accustomed to this. He called it "spitting up," and no one ever specifically asked him if he "spit up." To Pete, vomiting was something that happened when you were sick, and he wasn't sick.

Once this problem was identified and the medical team convinced Pete that this was something that should be addressed, a work-up began. A modified barium swallow (MBS) was performed. This showed that he had severe problems of the esophagus, which did not let all his food into his stomach. Instead, some came up again and some went into his lungs; consequently, pneumonia followed. If things continued like this, Pete would likely continue to experience one respiratory infection after another, with continuing debilitation and progressive weight loss. As well, the germs causing the pneumonias would get stronger with the development of antibiotic resistance. Pete was offered a feeding tube as an alternate way of getting nutrition.

Pete led a simple life with his wife, and there was no reason he couldn't go on with a feeding tube. His lungs were likely to improve if the food material was stopped from entering. He would gain weight and strength if more food found its way to his stomach. This was a simple enough procedure, and he tolerated it well. His wife was taught the day-to-day use of the feeding tube, which is a pretty straightforward task, and how to troubleshoot and identify signs of impending problems. The homecare nurses supported them, and together Pete did very well at home, gaining weight, strength, and vitality.

Pete's story reminds us of the problems that can arise with a "don't ask, don't tell" approach to physical well-being. It also shows the dangers of accepting as "normal" issues that, once properly identified, could quite easily be addressed. In Pete's case, it turned out that he was an excellent candidate for a feeding tube, which addressed his respiratory infections and weight loss and thus allowed him to regain his health and strength.

Healthcare providers can help elders sort out if what they consider to be "normal" is healthy or not. Both patients and providers need to be prepared to discuss delicate or unpleasant topics.

CARE AND COMFORT

Care and comfort is a broad term that covers a lot of territory. It is a common approach with the elderly, as well as a goal for long-term care. When plans are based on the "care and comfort" approach, day-to-day quality of life is the main focus.

A "care and comfort" plan can be implemented anywhere along the timeline. Sometimes, elderly patients have this philosophy well established and well thought out. This is especially true for ancient ones who feel they still have a lot of living to do and want to *live* life rather than *prolong* it or be bothered by unpleasant medical care.

Other times, there is a particular event that prompts patients to adopt "care and comfort" as their new direction for health care. For example, a stroke, a major infection, or the identification of a catastrophic diagnosis can lead elders to reevaluate goals and approaches. In some of these circumstances, the ancient ones cannot provide their consent or cannot comprehend the decision-making process or any of the procedures being considered. In these cases, decisions will need to be made by a healthcare agent, based on advance directives (if they exist) and/or the patients' best interests. In the case of some new diagnoses that prompt a "care and comfort" approach, terminal care may even be the next step. The overall life expectancy may be so short that it may not justify even a brief episode of the unpleasantness that can come with medical interventions.

"Care and comfort" may also be the best approach when there are preexisting conditions such as advanced dementia, end-stage heart disease, or lung disease, which so negatively affect the quality of life that any other approach would seem unkind. At times, there is the possibility that medical care is really prolonging a death and not a life.

"Comfort measures only" is an approach to care that is taken when the goal shifts from a diagnostic and treatment mode to a supportive plan. This is a plan that can forfeit medical work-up of a complaint or problem based upon degree of difficulty. As some of the earlier examples have shown, at this stage, identification of causes of problems ("know the unknown") may be deferred to minimize discomfort with the idea that more information would not change the plan of care ("find it, fix it"). There is also avoidance of treatments that have the goal of prolonging life for the sake of length of life. At this point, the patient's situation may include a level of discomfort on a daily basis, a disdain for the loss of function of independence, and/or despair at the thought of things getting worse. Coupled with the frequent loss of significant others, it can hardly be surprising that so many people tell me they're "ready to go."

"Care and comfort" does not preclude treatment for any of the more minor problems that pop up along the way, such as infections or other problems that are simple to treat. More serious problems may be treated with the simplest option of care. The "care and comfort " approach focuses on just that—treatment that is aimed to make the patient comfortable and is simply centered around the thoughtfulness that accompanies any decision regarding medical options.

Flo

Flo was only in her early seventies. However, she suffered from a fairly typical form of Alzheimer's disease. Her devoted husband was very involved in her care. He kept her at home until she began having the typical "sundowning" behaviors so characteristic of Alzheimer's disease, including wandering and bouts of rage and agitation that increased in the afternoon and at night.

Flo's medical care was uneventful for much of the three years she had been living on the dementia unit. She was on anti-psychotic medications, which controlled her difficult behaviors quite effectively. These meds, however, contributed to weight gain and the subsequent development of diabetes. She loved to eat, and sweets were one of her greatest pleasures. Her family did not want the healthcare team to withhold these favorite foods. Her comfort and contentment was the very most important thing to the family.

Out of the blue, Flo developed weakness and severe and sudden shortness of breath. She was admitted to the community hospital, where she became acutely agitated and unable to cooperate with the usual medical care. She fiercely defended herself against blood draws, pulled out tubes, and spit out oral medication. The medical team needed to tie her hands to keep her from pulling out the IV.

While Flo was in the hospital, they determined that she had blood loss from the GI tract. Eventually, after receiving sufficient sedation, she tolerated her IV long enough to receive two units of blood. This perked her up so that she had more strength, and she began fighting off the hospital staff with even more vigor.

Normally, a work-up (blood tests, x-rays, and/or "scope" tests) would have been scheduled to identify where, why, and how serious the bleeding was. However, to pursue either the "know the unknown" or "find it, fix it" approach, Flo would have needed to be sedated and likely physically and chemically restrained. Even though the goal had always been "care and comfort," now that her providers were faced with a diagnostic dilemma, the plan needed to be reviewed, explaining actual risks of forgoing a work-up.

Flo's husband and her physician agreed that the risks of pursuing a diagnosis outweighed the benefit. Her distress and total inability to comprehend any part of the plan or procedures made it unwise to continue down the diagnostic road. They also decided that there would be no more transfusions after seeing the distress it had caused.

Flo returned to her nursing home at her baseline level of comfort and activity. Still pleasantly confused, she strolled around the unit patting and kissing her favorite people when she saw them. This status quo continued for a year or so.

Her dementia progressed. As she continued with worsening cognitive status and little intelligible speech, her nonverbal cues provided the only clues to the specifics of her problems. Her appetite was off, activity slowed down, and her color was very pale. She also suffered from weight loss, intermittent agitation, apparent nausea, and abdominal pain. She was treated for each symptom in turn.

Unfortunately, at times such as weekends, the regular staff were sometimes replaced with on-call nurses or doctors, some of whom would question the overall plan and order blood work. The results would show abnormal levels, such as anemia, but that had already been made evident by the blood in her stools. Each time tests were ordered and new results received, the discussion of whether or not to proceed with additional diagnostic tests began again. Time after time, Flo's frustrated husband restated the goal for her care: to avoid agitating his wife (which even the simplest medical procedures invariably did) and to ensure that she remained comfortable.

Despite the detours that threatened to occur whenever new practitioners intervened, in general the "care and comfort" approach worked well for Flo. Controlling her diet eased her discomfort, as did pain medication. Some days, she would actually seem like her old self.

Over time, however, Flo continued to decline, and those who knew and loved her found it hard to see her weaken. She could not enjoy her food, and she lost weight. Her good days became fewer and farther between. Her bad days required medication to get her through. Hospice came in to support Flo, her husband, and the staff. In the end, she died in the nursing home where she had lived for nearly five years, cared for by the staff who knew her well, with her husband at her side.

Flo's story shows us that even with a well-established goal of comfort measures only, it is easier to maintain this approach during times of relative wellness. It is easier to let the diabetic eat cake than to decide not to give a transfusion for blood loss or to treat the latest of several infections. Providers can become so entrenched in the traditional "find it, fix it" approach that it sometimes requires strenuous effort to get them to deviate from that bias and allow for symptomatic and supportive treatment. I have seen times when family members are perceived in a bad light or are even considered villainous for trying to uphold this approach.

Fortunately, I think times are changing and there is more acceptance of the "care and comfort" approach to healthcare. In this way, the comfort measures at end of life have parallels to the natural childbirth movement. The new thinking focuses on treating death as a natural event that should be allowed to occur in a peaceful environment and to be free of unnecessary medical intervention. I strongly expect that in the days ahead we will see increasing support for these types of choices.

* * *

As the stories in this chapter have shown, the approaches discussed here will come into play whether ancient ones and their families are dealing with chronic aches and pains or end-of-life care. In each case, "the plan" to address the issues must first take into account the goals and the approach to the problem or situation at hand. Then the next part to consider is the actual implementation of the plan.

In the chapters that follow, my assumption is that the primary goal for the ancient ones is to remain in or return to their home. With this in mind, Chapter 3 looks at the mostly functional issues in maintaining a safe at-home plan.

Chapter Three

Home Sweet Home: Safety Measures

This chapter is focused on the issues and challenges that elders of advanced age face as they try to maintain a safe, comfortable, and functional life in their own home. For those who are able to remain in their home, independence is a goal, but even ancient ones who are fairly healthy often require assistance of various kinds to support this situation. This chapter offers suggestions for changes that may be needed to update the home situation and to address potential risks before big problems develop.

The following section starts with a general discussion of overall safety measures and precautions that friends and family can take to help the elders avoid harm. Next, we'll take a more specific look at some of the functional types of issues that impact the daily lives of ancient ones who live at home—including difficult topics of smoking, drinking, and driving—and what can be done to help them continue to live independently. Finally, we will identify the types of physical and sensory changes that affect many ancient ones, so caregivers can make adjustments as necessary to keep them safe at home.

Wallet-Sized Record of Vital Information

One very important thing to do for overall safety of a frail elder is to provide a way for them to keep vital information such as names and phone numbers of important people with them at all times. This includes next of kin, healthcare agent (if not the same), and primary care provider. If there is a MOLST form, place it on a wallet-sized card and keep it with the elder's identification papers. It should also be clearly visible in the home, such as on the fridge or near the phone.

An organization called the File of Life Foundation (www.folife.org) has created a useful card that lets users list emergency information in a standardized format. Be sure to include important medical conditions or allergies. You may also want to add an updated list of current medications, but this is advised *only if you can keep the list updated.*

A Few Words About Emergency Buttons

For everyday emergencies, emergency service retailers such as Lifeline offer safety equipment that provide an emergency button that will summon a rescue squad when activated during a medical emergency. These devices are usually worn either in the style of a wristwatch or a pendant. In theory, this is a great plan. However, in order for this system to be effective, the elderly person must actually

1. wear the device;

2. be able to use it properly.

If you do decide to take this route, be sure to pick a system that's easy for the senior to use. In particular, the emergency buttons should be large and easy enough for the senior to see and press, with no complicated added steps. Since many accidents happen in the bathroom, the device should also be waterproof—and the elder should be reminded to keep it on even during a shower or bath.

As technology advances there will be improvements in these safety devices. There already is a version that automatically summons help when a sudden drop in elevation is detected during a fall.

Safeguards Against Falls

As seniors age, many areas of physical decline can predispose them to falls. These potentially dangerous challenges include

- loss of physical strength, flexibility, equilibrium, and/or balance;

- slower reflexes;

- impaired vision;

- sluggish circulation;

- diminished breathing capacity;

- pain with walking;

- weakness that affects stability of gait; and

- improper footwear.

These age-related changes, combined with medical problems (and their associated medications), are a setup for falls, which are often catastrophic in the elderly. This is especially true for those with weakened bones (osteoporosis) and thinning skin.

In fact, among older adults, falls are the leading cause of both fatal and nonfatal injuries—many of which lead to hospitalizations and subsequent institutionalization. In 2012, emergency departments treated approximately 2.4 million nonfatal falls among older adults, and more than 722,000 of these patients needed to be hospitalized.[1]

Broken bones (fractures) are a common and problematic occurrence in the very old. Big falls, little falls—and sometimes no fall or trauma of any kind—can result in fractures. Some require simple splinting or casting, while others need surgical repair; all need time to heal. A cast on the forearm is not a big deal in a younger person, but older people may have their delicate balance thrown off, which can prevent them from being able to walk on their own or manage daily activities until it has fully healed. Other common injuries are rib and pelvic fractures. These are painful, and the broken bones cannot be fully stabilized. This creates mobility issues and increases the risk for other problems, such as infection and pain-related complications.

Hip fractures are usually surgically repaired and often end up with a variety of complicating issues. Elders with weaker and/or more cognitively impaired baseline conditions often experience subsequent problems. People do recover, but they usually suffer a host of complications, including pain and side effects from pain medications; mental status changes; urinary retention; urinary tract infections (UTIs); pneumonia; and the worsening of chronic medical problems.

Many fractures require a limitation of weight-bearing status, which refers to the ability to use the affected area during the healing process. Surprisingly, it is not uncommon to have no restriction after a hip fracture, meaning that the patient can walk without learning a new way to walk. However, other fractures may require no weight or just a little amount of weight on the limb. This can be very problematic in the recovery process. A frail, weak, and/or confused person will have difficulty with managing these restrictions. Rehab will be needed to regain strength, endurance, and gait stability. Recovery is often not in a straight line, with progress intertwined with setbacks.

---

[1] Centers for Disease Control and Prevention, National Center for Injury Prevention and Control. Web–based Injury Statistics Query and Reporting System (WISQARS) [online]. Accessed August 15, 2013.

The good news is that there are ways to prevent many of these accidents. Strategies are aimed at

- maintaining or improving physical well-being;

- using adaptive equipment;

- avoiding dangerous apparatus such as ladders or power tools;

- modifying the environment by rearranging the living space; and/or

- adding the assistance of another person.

Let's take a look at some of the specific safeguards that can be put in place to help prevent falls.

ADEQUATE FITNESS

The best safeguard against falling is maintaining a general level of adequate fitness. This involves

- regular physical activity;

- exercises for strength endurance and balance;

- adequate sleep and/or compensation for lack of prolonged nighttime sleep with naps throughout the day;

- proper nutrition, regular meals, and nutritious snacks;

- good healthcare, regular medical visits, and proper medication use; and

- a safe environment that has been adapted to changing needs.

Even a modest exercise program can yield benefits in terms of fitness. "If you don't use it, you lose it" is an age-old adage that is especially true. Regular exercise also

- decreases anxiety and improves symptoms of depression;

- increases length and quality of sleep;

- improves regularity with bowel functioning;

- reduces high blood pressure;

- maintains blood sugar levels more effectively; and

- improves cardiac health and circulation to hands and feet.

The use of light weights is a valuable way to improve overall strength. A physical therapist or trainer who has expertise with the elderly can set up an exercise program that seniors can follow at home, in a gym, or at a senior center. The program should be tailored to the individual's need and have a doctor's approval.

Movement exercises, such as yoga and Tai Chi, can also help improve balance and improve stability, in addition to promoting a sense of calm. These exercises are gentle enough for the elderly and can be learned at any age. A walking program is another simple way to improve fitness for those who are currently steady on their feet.

CANES, WALKERS, AND WHEELCHAIRS

For some ancient ones, even the simple act of walking around, or *ambulation,* can be a difficult and hazardous activity. It requires strength, balance, motor planning, and judgment. The elderly need physical capabilities to get around and negotiate obstacles in their path, in addition to performing the activities of daily living (ADLs), bathing, dressing, and meal preparation.

Many ancient ones often need assistive devices, such as walkers and canes, to take steps. These are simple interventions that can improve stability and minimize the risk of falling. (Crutches also keep weight off a leg, but most elderly people do not do well with these, finding them more cumbersome than the alternatives.) The primary care provider can order a consultation with a physical or occupational therapist, who will perform evaluations for these devices and set up an exercise program.

These devices need to be fitted for size (and checked for soundness if pulled out of storage or borrowed from a neighbor's cousin). Canes provide support for those unsteady on their feet. Walkers provide more support for those with balance and weakness problems. Both walkers and canes help offload the weight from weakened or painful weight-bearing joints, such as hips and knees. However, since the weight is then shifted to the upper extremities, elders also need to take care to prevent injury to shoulders, elbows, and wrists.

Neither canes nor walkers work very well if used improperly. Walkers are especially troublesome because they require two hands to use, leaving no hands free to carry the tea to the table. To address these challenges, walker baskets and trays, which fasten to the front of the walker, can be used to transport the mail and other lightweight items (although certainly not hot tea!). In addition, walkers can be fitted with wheels or skis, depending on the type of floor surfaces and the skills and strength of the user.

Wheelchairs are great inventions but take skill, strength (either the sitter's or the pusher's), and space to make them useful. In fact, many ambulatory people choose to use wheelchairs for long distances, such as shopping malls or long household distances. However, elders who are unable to bear weight on their feet must figure out how to transfer from bed to wheelchair and on and off the toilet. If the senior has sufficient upper body strength or a transfer slide board, then this can be done independently; however, if more assistance is needed, then the elder can use a mechanical lift to improve safety and general ease.

MODIFICATIONS FOR INDOOR AND OUTDOOR LIVING SPACES

It's also helpful to modify the ancient one's living space to promote safety. Many times a physical and/or an occupational therapist can conduct a home safety evaluation and provide specific recommendations for the elder's situation. Some ways to eliminate obstacles in the person's environment include minimizing the accumulation of objects in the pathways. Trash, materials to be recycled, and generalized clutter are tripping hazards and should be removed from the living space and passageways as often as needed to prevent peril. Trash removal is a task that is good to delegate, if possible, since it can be hazardous for an elderly person to carry bulky bags when walking through doors, across thresholds, and up and down stairs and outside. Similarly, it can be difficult for elders to carry a basket of laundry back and forth to the washer and dryer.

Good lighting is essential for a safe environment, and this is not an area to compromise. Older eyes let less light in, so the living space needs to be brightly lit. The switches should be accessible (located in entrances to rooms) so there is no need for fumbling (or stumbling) about in the dark. A light that turns on with a clap of the hands can be a fun addition, though not as a primary light source. Nightlights are very sensible for those who need to make trips to the bathroom during the night. Remember to change the bulbs throughout the house before the elderly person finds the stepstool, climbs up, and then falls down. This also applies to batteries that need to be changed in smoke and carbon monoxide detectors, which should always be installed and kept in good working order.

Rugs should be secured firmly to the floor (or removed). Always try to avoid scatter rugs, which can bunch up and get caught on walkers, canes, and shuffling feet. If the ancient ones simply love their rugs to the point where they insist on keeping them, make sure the rugs have

DEALING WITH RESISTANCE

While modifying the home environment can be a key to keeping elders safe at home, some seniors are reluctant to accept help, make changes, or allow you to make changes. The following tips have been adapted from the Mayo Clinic's website to help families prevent or work through the elder's resistance.

Determine what help is needed. Evaluate what kind of help the senior needs and which changes might work best.

Talk about it when everyone is relaxed. This will make it easier for everyone to share their thoughts, preferences, and even objections in a calm way that leaves the subject open for discussion.

Ask about the ancient one's preferences. Elders are more likely to accept help if they have some input into the changes. If necessary, simplify your explanations and the decisions you expect the senior to make.

Pick your battles. Consider the elder's point of view and focus on the big picture. Ignore minor issues that don't really affect care.

Suggest a trial run to test the waters. Agree in advance that if the change isn't effective, you'll reverse it.

Emphasize that the change should prolong independence. Remind elders that you are trying to help them stay at home for as long as possible.

Ask family members and friends to help. This makes the issues less personal, and friends and family might be able to help you persuade your loved one to accept help.

Don't give up. If the ancient one doesn't want to discuss the topic the first time you bring it up, try again later.

Enlist the help of a professional. If seniors continue to resist changes that are required for their safety, ask their doctor to speak with them. They may be more willing to listen to the advice of a professional.

Source: Adapted from *www.mayoclinic.org/healthy-living/caregivers/in-depth/caring-for-the-elderly/art-20048403?pg=2*

skid-proof pads. Thick pile rugs are good in case of a fall, but in some cases they may actually precipitate a fall because of the depth of the pile.

Handrails are very useful additions to many areas of a home, especially if the walkers and canes are not consistently used in the home. "Furniture walking" is a common strategy used by elders. Instead of using the cane or walker, the senior negotiates moving through the house by holding on to the chair, the table, the bookcase, and so forth. This strategy is only effective if the objects are solid and don't move, rock, or have wheels.

The outside environment poses many safety challenges as well. For many people, outdoor work has always been part of their ADLs. This can include yard work, gardening, and snow shoveling. These activities may be part chore, part hobby, and part habit. However, there comes a time when continuing these activities goes beyond reason, though it may still be hard to get the elders to stop. I have seen family members pave the garden in an attempt to help their elderly loved ones, only to see container gardens sprout up elsewhere.

Hypothermia and Overheating

The most obvious dangerous weather often occurs in winter. Extreme cold, snow, and ice are very hazardous for the elderly. Falls and hypothermia are seasonal threats for people living in the northern climates. Hypothermia, or low body temperature, can happen quickly in a snow bank, but it can also occur in a home with the heat set too low. Confusion can be either a cause or a symptom of hypothermia.

This is not the time for pride but rather caution. Bring a cane—or better yet a strong arm—for elderly people to hold on to if they must venture outdoors in the winter. Long coats that extend to the knees or beyond offer double protection: they are extra warm and also act as a cushion in the event of a fall. However, no safety measure is meant to do away with common sense when the reasonable action is to just stay indoors. A game of bridge in bad weather is not worth a broken hip no matter how good the partner is or how severe the cabin fever.

Extreme heat is also dangerous for the elderly. They must take care to avoid heat stroke and dehydration. Air conditioning cools and dehumidifies the air, improving both comfort and breathing in those with respiratory troubles. Remaining in an indoor, cool environment is one of the best options for managing the severe heat. When this is not possible, make sure that elders adjust fluid intake and activity level. Frequent cold or ice drinks help keep down the heat, though elders should take care to not overdo the sweets found in soda or other sugary beverages.

Elders with a compromised cardiac or respiratory system may have trouble with fluids and may need specific advice about coping with the heat. These people should consult their primary care physicians. Otherwise, they should drink eight to twelve glasses of cold or cool beverages throughout the day—more if there is a lot of sweating.

During hot weather, elders may wish to avoid hot meals to prevent adding to the heat, not only in the body but also in the room. Cooking with a microwave or using a slow cooker will prevent adding more heat to the kitchen.

It's important to note that many elderly people feel chilly even on a warm day and may still feel this way even in extreme heat. Even so, have them take their sweaters off so they don't overheat. Ancient ones also need sunscreen when outdoors to prevent burns, which can quickly become severe for those with thinning skin.

Weather Emergency Plans

An elder living alone is particularly vulnerable in a weather emergency, be that a snowstorm, hurricane, tornado, or thunderstorm. Loss of power, water, and/or heat can lead to catastrophe. Make sure the elderly person has emergency equipment, such as

- flashlights with fresh batteries (spare batteries can be difficult for elders to replace, especially in the dark);

- battery-operated wall lights with light sensors;

- extra water, in bottles that are small enough for the elders to lift and pour from easily;

- blankets, in a place they can reach;

- nonperishable foods, and a way to open them;

- medications, with clear directions; and

- first aid supplies that the elders know how and when to use effectively.

Emergency generators can also be helpful if the elders can manage these devices on their own (as in flip a switch) or have neighbors who will help them. As in all situations, cognitive impairment can turn challenges into a crisis. Whenever possible, arrange for neighbors to check in on shut-ins when the weather keeps others away.

In situations that involve a prolonged power outage (more than twenty-four hours), even a fairly capable elderly person should not be alone, and arrangements will need to be made for safer shelter, such as a brief stay with a relative or in a nursing home. These situations can quickly turn into a crisis, so it is essential to create an emergency plan well ahead of time.

Smoking, Alcohol Consumption, and Driving

Three very big issues in the discussion of safety are smoking, alcohol consumption, and driving. While all of these situations may need to be broached delicately, changing habits can be a major key in keeping elders safe.

SMOKING

Aside from the serious consequences to the elder's heart and lungs, smoking is also dangerous in terms of fire safety; these risks are increased by the effects of advanced age. In particular, the risk of uncontrolled fire increases with cognitive impairment, poor reflexes, less-than-nimble fingers, sedating medicines, and decreased sense of smell. It is a good idea to check the elder's clothing for burn holes, just to see if there is a problem.

Medical advice will always be to stop smoking or cut down, but at this point with a very old person who chooses to smoke, supervision or even a flame-retardant bib may be an effective compromise. In some cases the elders may accept an electronic cigarette instead of a traditional one. I even had a patient who chose to hold a straw like a cigarette, and it seemed to produce her desired effect.

ALCOHOL CONSUMPTION

In addition to drinking for pleasure, some elders use alcohol to self-treat issues like loneliness, boredom, and depression. Unfortunately, alcohol consumption presents a huge problem related to safety. Whether seniors drink beer, wine, whiskey, or another liquor, their tolerance for it will decrease with advanced age. In fact, as age progresses, the effects of inebriation increase. In addition to the physical problems associated with heavy alcohol use, such as maladies of the stomach and liver, falls are much more common when elders are "walking under the influence."

Regular alcohol consumption also greatly increases the risk of delirium when a medical event prompts a hospitalization because the elders begin to suffer from "alcohol abstinence syndrome." Basically, when regular consumers of alcohol are suddenly unable to drink, they may experience a whole series of symptoms, including irritability, anxiety, hallucinations, and even seizures. In some of these cases, the effects are not related as much to the amount of alcohol consumed as they are to the regularity of use. As such, even the habit of one daily drink over thirty years can cause trouble for ancient ones, who suddenly experience mental status changes when medical illness intercedes. Due to the risks of regular alcohol drinking, the best advice is to limit intake to one drink daily. However, if there are medical problems or medications that impair thinking or balance, truly none is better.

DRIVING

The decision of when to ensure that the elderly person surrenders the driving license (and actually stops driving) can be a tough call. In our society, where self-determination and independence is so very valued, the loss of a driver's license is monumental. Everyone has places to go: to the doctor, shopping, to visit friends, out to lunch, or just out for a drive. For those who still drive, it is freedom manifested.

Unfortunately, families often act as enablers long past the time when elders should stop driving. In their view, as long as seniors still drive, it limits the number of tasks other family members need to take on themselves, so they allow it even though they know it's dangerous. For instance, I have seen family members support an elder's wish to keep driving, but then refuse to allow that same elder to drive with the grandchildren in the car. This makes little sense. If seniors are not safe enough drivers for the children, why would they be safe to drive alone? If they are at risk of backing into another car that contains someone else's children, is this still acceptable?

The physical and cognitive skills required in driving are numerous, and aging affects them all. From vision and hearing loss, to slowing reflexes and poor mobility in the neck, none of these physical problems are as hard to identify as the cognitive decline that indicates it is no longer safe for the ancient one to drive.

In an ideal situation, the ancient one will have some insight about the declining functioning and volunteer to hand over the keys. When that is not the case, then families need to get involved. One indicator that it's time for elders to stop driving is when they get lost when navigating through a previously familiar area. If there is dispute about driving capabilities, the senior can take an objective test at the Registry of Motor Vehicles or some other entity, such as an acute rehab facility. I have even seen families disable the car by pulling out the spark plugs, hiding keys to prevent driving, or requesting a police officer to follow the driver to evaluate competency.

Compensations for Diminished Senses

We all rely on our senses to keep us aware, safe, and connected to each other. However, while all the years may add wisdom, they are also likely to diminish the senses. Some of the most common and difficult changes associated with age are the loss of vision, hearing, smell, taste, and touch. At times, accommodations must be made with adaptive equipment and increased help in the home to compensate for these changes. This is likely to be an evolving situation that needs more help as time goes on. As you read the following sections, keep in mind that often elders have not just one of these problems but several—or even all.

VISION

Close vision begins to decline in our forties and continues to deteriorate over several decades. This happens with most people, even those who previously had 20/20 or excellent distance vision. In general, for close reading, this type of defect can be corrected with over-the-counter magnifying or reading glasses. However, elders with vision problems for distance need prescription glasses. Seniors who experience a loss of clarity in both near and far vision may actually need bifocals.

As you work to support the ancient ones, make sure prescriptions are up to date and glasses are kept clean. The ability to see and interpret their surroundings also helps elderly people to prevent falls. Note that bifocals can complicate matters, because they require the viewer to look through a certain part of the lens for a particular activity. Simple things, such as going up or down stairs, can become problematic with bifocals.

In addition to normally reduced vision from aging, there are also many medical issues that compromise vision. The prevalence of glaucoma, cataracts, macular degeneration, and diabetic eye disorders is reason to have good eye care. These problems require regular appointments, which can lead to transportation issues, and may result in a complicated schedule of eye drops.

Visual impairment complicates all aspect of life. Some examples include

- activities of daily living (ADLs) (e.g., struggles with bathing, dressing, toileting);

- safety (e.g., increased risk of falls and other mishaps);

- independence (e.g., inability to see well enough to drive);

- medication management (e.g., unable to read instructions and labels); and

- recreation and socialization (e.g., unable to read the numbers on bingo cards or bowling scores).

For those with reduced visual function, simplifying the environment with decluttering can promote safety. There are numerous devices to help visually impaired persons maintain independence, such a talking clocks or specialized appliances. Your state's commission for the blind is a good resource for learning what is available.

When encountering a person with visual impairment it is imperative to identify yourself and your reason for being there. This should be the norm for health care providers with all patients; however, everyone should do this with the visually impaired. This prevents confusion or awkwardness in social interactions because everyone wants to know exactly who they are talking to.

HEARING

Hearing loss is common in advanced age. As you communicate with ancient ones who have experienced a decline in hearing, remind yourself that verbal information may not be well understood. To avoid mix-ups, write down things such as medication adjustments, appointments, and other important information. Make sure the writing is clearly done in big enough and dark enough print.

Some elderly people who experience a decline in hearing start to withdraw from others and self-isolate due to the discouragement and frustration they experience from missing out on conversations. For these people, one-on-one conversations may be better than group discussions. Be sure to minimize distracting sounds, turn off the music or TV, and face the listener while speaking clearly to aid communication.

Fortunately, there is much that can be done. Even for those with limited hearing, music can bring back happy memories and improve mood. Singing and making music—even clapping or drumming—show positive effects on those suffering from dementia. Hearing aides are getting better all the time. As well, more devices are built with hearing loss in mind, from shake-awake alarm clocks to close-captioned television and amplified telephones.

SMELL

The sense of smell is diminished in the elderly, which means they may struggle to identify important things such as smoke, gas, or spoiled food.

To help the ancient ones who remain at home, friends and family can keep an eye (and nose!) on the contents of the refrigerator. Use a Sharpie pen to date disposable food containers and leftovers. Otherwise, elders may miss the tiny print of the expiration date, and their nose may not reliably perform the "sniff test."

In some cases, it may also become necessary to discuss housekeeping or personal grooming. For instance, an elderly person may not notice unpleasant environmental smells or even their own body odor, which may be highly obvious to visitors. This may be an indication that assistance is needed for the tasks of housework or bathing. This situation may require a delicate but necessary conversation.

Sometimes it's the absence of smell that is all that's needed. Help take out the trash, clean the litter box, or even just open the window and bring in the fresh air to chase out the stuffiness.

TASTE

Taste is another sense that can lose its acuity with age progression, and certain medical conditions and medications can cause a persistent bad taste or dryness in the mouth. Therefore, it's important to make foods for ancient ones as appealing as possible. Adding moisture to foods in the form of gravies and sauces can be beneficial. Offering soup rather than a sandwich can make a meal more appetizing. When goals of care are liberal and dietary restrictions are few (or lifted), adding butter or cream to foods can improve the palatability of meals, especially if the ancient ones are trying to combat undesirable weight loss.

Fragrances also have the power to soothe and can stimulate appetites for elders who still have a good sense of smell. The smell of baking bread, simmering stew, or chocolate chip cookies can be used to improve interest in meals. Some of the simple olfactory experiences can trigger memories, and it makes sense to capitalize on this.

At the same time, it's essential to make sure that elders don't overcompensate for weak taste buds by adding too much salt. (Note also that salt is often an issue with prepackaged or processed foods, which elders may tend to purchase because they're easy to prepare.) This warning is particularly important for elders with a tendency to retain fluids, especially those with congestive heart failure.

TOUCH

Many elderly people suffer from *neuropathy*, which refers to distortion in the sense of touch. It causes decreased, unpleasant, or painful sensations in the hands and feet and may be brought on by medical conditions such as diabetes, vitamin B12 deficiency, or poor circulation.

Neuropathy puts ancient ones at risk for injury because they can't feel the danger until it's too late. For instance, they may not detect the pebble in the shoe until a blister forms, or they may scald their feet because they can't detect how hot the water actually is.

When elders suffer from this condition, extra caution is advised to help them avoid injury. Well fitting and supportive shoes with socks are advised, and barefoot walking is discouraged. Be sure they examine their feet for blisters, cuts, or infections on a regular basis (this is especially important for diabetics). A long-handled mirror may help with this activity. In the home, set the temperature of the water heater no higher than 120°F; water for a bath should be closer to 100°F to prevent scald injuries.

The emotional aspects of touch are also a key component to the ancient one's health and wellness. There have been new discussions in the medical community about touch—and the lack of it—and how it affects individuals. It has long been known about the deleterious effect of touch deprivation in children. It stands to reason that all humans can benefit from physical contact and touch. Yet many of these elderly persons are socially isolated. Consequently, the addition of human touch can be another important aspect of keeping them happy and well. Things like pets, massages, hugs, or even a two-handed handshake may help someone feel happier and more alive.

ELDER ABUSE

Elder abuse can affect men and women of all ethnic backgrounds and social status. The following types of abuse are commonly accepted as the major categories of elder mistreatment:

Physical Abuse—Inflicting, or threatening to inflict, physical pain or injury on a vulnerable elder, or depriving them of a basic need.

Emotional Abuse—Inflicting mental pain, anguish, or distress on an elder person through verbal or nonverbal acts.

Sexual Abuse—Nonconsensual sexual contact of any kind; coercing an elder to witness sexual behaviors.

Exploitation—Illegal taking, misuse, or concealment of funds, property, or assets of a vulnerable elder.

Neglect—Refusal or failure by those responsible to provide food, shelter, healthcare, or protection for a vulnerable elder.

Abandonment—The desertion of a vulnerable elder by anyone who has assumed the responsibility for care or custody of that person.

Domestic elder abuse generally refers to any of the above types of mistreatment that are committed by someone with whom the elder has a special relationship (for example, a spouse, sibling, child, friend, or caregiver).

Institutional abuse generally refers to any of the above types of mistreatment occurring in residential facilities (such as a nursing home, assisted living facility, group home, board and care facility, foster home, etc.) and is usually perpetrated by someone with a legal or contractual obligation to provide some element of care or protection.

All states have adult protective and long-term care ombudsman programs, family care supports, and home and community care services that can help older adults with activities of daily living. Call the Eldercare Locator at **800-677-1116** for information and referrals on services in your area. Report any concerns about elder abuse or neglect to any healthcare provider.

Source: National Center on Elder Abuse. Administration on Aging. Department of Health and Human Services. www.ncea.aoa.gov

Chapter Four

Activities of Daily Living (ADLs)
Up, Dressed, and Looking Good

As families take steps to help the very old remain in their own homes, it is wise to expect that there is or will be a decline in self-care. Whether they need help with driving, snow shoveling, bill paying (financially or administratively), or handling more basic issues of personal care, the age-related changes are often subtle. Sometimes, observant friends and families note these changes but are not sure how and when to intervene. Ancient ones may also have different priorities about which tasks to hold on to and which to delegate. Their ability to continue to meet their own needs will depend upon an assortment of physical and cognitive skills, financial resources, and social support.

Working with the assumption that independence and safety are the general goals, let's start by examining the ups and downs of daily life. Activities of daily living or ADLs, is the term used to describe the tasks involved in personal care. These tasks include

- dressing;

- bathing;

- toileting;

- homemaking (or housekeeping);

- shopping;

- money management;

- meal planning and preparation; and

- medication management.

Numerous physical problems may limit the management of ADLs. For instance, many medical conditions, and/or their treatments, cause generalized fatigue. Other problems, like arthritis and other musculoskeletal problems, are common among ancient ones and can be disabling. Pain in the big joints—such as the spine, hips, and knees—can dramatically impair mobility and set up the need to meet with the primary care physician for a pain management plan so that pain and/or poor mobility do not lead to a decreased quality of life.

Range of motion (the ability to bend and straighten joints) diminishes with arthritic changes, which can also make daily activities difficult. Weight gain and depression can follow immobility. Stiffness in the hips and knees can make it difficult to bend over to put on socks and shoes. Cutting toenails can be out of the question, and if the elder has poor eyesight, problems with feet may go undetected.

The little joints of the hands and fingers can experience pain and stiffness, which cause problems in dressing and other fine-motor skills. Elders often experience a loss of dexterity in these fine movements, which are needed to manage buttons and shoelaces, not to mention to open a pill bottle or frozen food package. One issue can quickly snowball into another, such as when the ancient one does not have the dexterity to replace a battery on a hearing aid.

Respiratory symptoms from heart or lung disease can drain the resources of elderly people to the point that even small tasks take all of their energy. Breathlessness can occur with activity, while improvement may occur with rest. If symptoms are severe, shortness of breath can limit even the ability to eat or speak. Conservation of energy and activity pacing involve a series of strategies that hold activities to a rate that gets the job done. These strategies include taking rest periods and planning activities, so that strenuous activities, such as laundry and shopping, are done during the freshest part of the day and not all in the same day. A simple change such as putting a chair in the bathroom or at the kitchen counter allows elders to sit instead of stand during chores and reduces overall fatigue. Otherwise, as the elders become tired during the course of the day, clumsiness may occur, with the increased likelihood of falling.

Cognitive impairment has huge implications for self-care, and changes in personal habits may be the earliest and clearest indicator of depression or dementia. The following discussion centers on the skills required for the various activities, and issues to look for to determine if the ancient one's needs are being met. Here, too, the focus remains on safety, problem identification, and strategies.

Basic Self-Care Tasks

Basic self-care tasks include dressing, bathing, and toileting. Let's take a closer look at the support that may be required for each.

DRESSING

As noted above, these various maladies can cause a lot of problems in getting dressed. Fortunately, elders and their families can help alleviate these problems by using creating thinking. Here are a few examples.

- If decreased movement in the shoulders makes pullovers impossible, try cardigans.
- If buttons are difficult for less-than-nimble fingers, try Velcro or zippers with a pull cord.
- Switch trousers with zippers to elastic-style pants (they don't all look like sweat suits).
- If laces are a challenge, fasten shoes with elastic laces that do not require tying, or change the style of shoe to something easier to put on, such as slip-ons.

There are catalogs of medical supplies that sell easy-to-wear clothing and adaptive equipment items that make life easier. These include all sorts of clever devices that are task-specific, from a button-holer (a device to assist with buttons) to a leg lifter (a device to help get the foot off the floor and into the bed).

Occupational therapists may serve as good resources for identifying the elder's functional limitations and developing a plan to improve the elder's performance status, suggest adaptive equipment, or rearrange the home environment to get the tasks done as easily and safely as possible. Talk to the ancient one's primary care provider to see if a referral for occupational therapy may be possible.

Families and friends should encourage elders to keep an open mind about making these changes in response to their shifting status. It may take a great deal of persuasion to convince the elder of the wisdom of changing either a long-standing behavior or a part of the habitual environment, but the reward of continued independence is often well worth it.

BATHING

Bathing is a national pastime in our society. We are a nation preoccupied with daily washing. However, today's elderly grew up and matured in the time when tubs were standard, and it was not that long ago that baths were weekly events. Showers are a relatively recent luxury, and many old people are not as comfortable with them.

The required frequency of bathing is much dependent upon the elders' activities of the day. An elderly person who is relatively inactive does not need a full bath or shower every day for the sake of cleanliness. The washing of hands, face, and privates are enough on a daily basis if the person is continent and not otherwise dirty. As noted earlier, the temperature of the water heater should be set no higher than 120°F, and a bath should be taken in water that's closer to 100°F to prevent scald injuries.

Tubs are great for soaking and limbering up stiff joints, but the ancient ones need to have enough flexibility to get in and out of them. This involves a deep knee bend from the ground on a slippery, hard, unforgiving surface. No wonder so many accidents occur here. To minimize risk, it's helpful to install handrails to as many points of contact as possible. *Never confuse a towel rack with a handrail.* A towel rack is designed to support a towel and not the weight of a person.

A solid vanity can provide stability but may take up too much space in a small bathroom. Consider a tub seat to prevent fatigue and the need for a deep knee bend. Some versions extend over the side of the tub to allow for a seated and stable transfer in and out of the tub.

Fit showers with sturdy grab bars to stabilize the ancient one's entrance to and exit from the shower. The floor of the shower should be clean (no soap scum), and it should have a nonskid surface. Slip-proof sandals may also prevent falls in the shower.

Shower chairs allow elders to sit down and are a good option if they are unsteady or have poor endurance. Shower chairs should be sturdy and waterproof. A hand-held sprayer added to the tub or shower can also be helpful, whether the elder uses it alone or with the help of an assistant.

Despite these safety precautions, there may come a time when the ancient one should avoid tubs and showers unless an attendant is present. Remember Grandma, who spent sixteen long hours on the floor of her tub, naked with the cold water dripping, because she didn't limit her baths to times when she wasn't alone in the house.

In some cases, it may be necessary to modify the bathroom or provide portable options for bathing instead. In particular, devices such as wheelchairs or walkers require a lot of space, and many home bathrooms just don't have enough room to accommodate them or the proper techniques to best use them.

Peri-Care

Peri-care (referring to the *perineum*, which is the area between the legs) is a term for the hygienic practices that occur after elimination. This is done independently for as long as possible, and when that is insufficient, an assistant is needed.

Peri-care is an essential and intimate task. It is common for the recipient of this care to feel deeply demoralized, and cognitively impaired individuals suffer distress during this aspect of care. Some family members may blanche at this level of care, and it may become necessary to hire a professional aide.

When incontinence occurs, there are no substitutions for thorough care. Caregivers should wear gloves and use warm water for each and every urine clean-up, whereas soap, followed by rinsing with warm water, is needed after each bowel movement. The last step of peri-care involves applying a layer of a barrier cream or ointment to protect the skin from the caustic next episode. There is a wide selection of barrier products available to maintain skin integrity. Almost any type of skin ointment that does not create irritation is fine to use, based on personal preference.

TOILETING

Toileting is the functional part of elimination. The danger is that when great urgency occurs in the need to get to the toilet, all safety measures will be discarded. Again the most important piece of this task is the elder's ability to recognize the body's need to go to the bathroom in the first place. Often, when "going to the bathroom," elders rush in, perform a complicated turn, and—possibly simultaneously—drop their underwear. Then there's the process of urination and moving of bowels. Straining can result in momentary changes in blood pressure and/or pulse. This can cause lightheadedness, dizziness, and falls. Next it's the paperwork, the reach and spinal twist, redressing, hand washing and drying, and the return to another room. This can be a very big job, and the successful completion of this necessary task is often a major limiting factor in independent living.

To help, consider raised toilet seats, which are molded plastic overlays. These minimize the deep knee bend necessary to use many toilets. Place a commode frame around the toilet to increase the height and provide firm and stable hand supports.

When the use of the bathroom is prohibitively difficult, the alternative is using a portable commode for toileting, and bathing at a washbasin. These portable options can make an improvised bathroom space where there was formerly a living room. Don't forget the antiseptic hand washing gel when there is no sink.

These plans will require another person to transport the contents of the commode and washbasin to and from the bathroom. The accumulation of wastes in a pot is distasteful for most people, even if diluted with water and covered with a lid. If you are the one assisting with this task, the use of latex gloves is advised along with frequent handwashing. A mask can be used if desired.

While men have the convenient option of using a urinal, the female urinals that currently exist are awkward and often not worth the trouble because spillage is common. Challenges such as urinary incontinence and constipation are discussed in Chapter 7.

Complex Self-Care Tasks

The decline or loss of higher-order tasks, such as shopping, driving, and money management, can have very serious consequences for ancient ones. An independent person may resist assistance in these areas until "something happens," such as an accident or a financial mishap. Again, paying attention to these issues before a crisis occurs can give warnings about problems in evolution.

DRIVING, ACCOUNTING, MEDICATION MANAGEMENT, AND HOUSEWORK

The basic strategy with these high-level tasks is simply delegation of duties. To address issues about driving, family members can volunteer to drive or hire a taxi service for outings. Money management includes not only bookkeeping, writing and mailing the checks to pay the bills, but also keeping track of the flow of money. If the family is unable to do so, then there may be the need to have a professional bookkeeper or bank pay the bills.

Medication management can be a big or small job depending upon the elder's medical condition. This task can be confusing in a medically complex senior and may require the oversight of a visiting nurse, in addition to a family member. This is discussed more extensively in Chapter 6.

Housework, including laundry, is one of the most commonly delegated tasks. If there are resources available, many seniors are willing to hand over this task in order to budget energy for more satisfying activities. Many communities offer housekeeping and shopping services for individuals with medical conditions that prevent them from completing those tasks. These services typically have sliding-scale fees based upon ability to pay.

If the ancient one is unwilling to delegate these tasks, as many people are reluctant to do, it may be useful to employ strategies for the elders to conserve energy so they can perform these chores later. This may require a deviation from lifelong patterns of ADLs, but most elders will agree that the price of independence is worth it.

MEAL PLANNING AND PREPARATION

Before we move on, let's take a closer look at one of the most important and frequently needed higher-order tasks: food preparation. Specifically, aging plays a huge role when it comes to food and all of the issues surrounding it:

- thinking about it (meal planning requires cognitive skills of insight, judgment, and memory);
- selecting it (this extends beyond knowing what is desired to finding it in a store and getting it in a cart);
- affording it (having the money either at hand or in the bank to buy the selected items);
- transporting it (getting it from store to kitchen);
- preparing it; and, finally, easy or hard,
- eating it.

These issues are complex, and the repercussions are far-reaching.

The most basic part of nutrition is recognizing the bodily sensation of hunger and putting that observation into action and finding food. This includes knowing how and when to shop, what to buy, managing the financial piece, getting the food home, and planning and preparing meals. The process between feeling hungry and putting food on the table requires a set of cognitive and physical skills, and lapses in any of the skills can have far-reaching consequences. Judgment enters the picture when deciding which food to buy and/or prepare. Insight into the ancient one's limitations will help in the delegation of duties. Limitations may be apparent to the elders, and they may ask for assistance. Family members or hired help may assume some of the responsibility for the various tasks of shopping and meal preparation.

Dementia and depression, both very common in the elderly, cloud judgment, impair skills, and set up risky situations. In fact, the ice cream in the cupboard or the toilet paper in the refrigerator may be a sign of cognitive decline. Spoiled food may remain in the fridge due to the elder's inability to read the small-print expiration dates or due to the ancient one's decreased sense of smell. Families may want to hire help to fill in the gaps, especially if they begin to notice problems with food storage and poor diet.

Other problems associated with poor diet, such as malnutrition with either weight loss or gain, may cause a propensity toward infection, decreased energy, and a host of other associated problems, including generalized debility. Social issues, such as boredom and isolation, can make mealtime for elders less than enjoyable, and cooking for one can seem not worth the effort. Congregate meal settings, such as lunch taken at a local senior center, can put camaraderie and enjoyment back into the dining experience.

Grocery Shopping

Consider all the physical challenges involved in the chore of grocery shopping. To be entirely independent, the ancient one must possess sufficient balance, strength, and endurance to get to and from the store, push the cart, reach and lift the items, see and read the labels, make appropriate food choices, and put items in the shopping cart before heading to the checkout counter. The groceries must then be lifted out of the cart onto the counter, and the shopper must have the money to pay for it. Then the shopper must transport the bags home (via car?), where they must be carried to the kitchen and put away. This can be an exhausting procedure and, for an elderly person, can easily take up an entire day's worth of energy. As well, elderly shoppers may make food choices based entirely on the lightness of packaging or location of food on the shelves, with the aim of avoiding products placed either too high or too low on the shelves.

Kitchen Navigation

Even if the shopping gets delegated and the food somehow ends up in the kitchen, dinner can remain a distant goal. Meal preparation is a complicated and tiring process, especially if the person relies on assistive devices, such as canes or walkers, or suffers from visual impairment or arthritic hands.

A major worry is the potential for fire when an elderly person with cognitive loss attempts to cook. Microwaves are safer alternatives to gas or electric stoves (which may need to be permanently shut off for safety). Choose appliances based upon the size of the control numbers, dials, and buttons, and the overall ease of use.

Within the kitchen, there may be changes necessary to accommodate advanced age. For example, it may make sense to consolidate daily use items to prevent unnecessary bending, reaching, and—God forbid—step-stool use. They may also forget to use items that aren't in plain sight. Yet elders may be considerably resistant to change.

Healthy, Balanced Diets

Elderly people benefit from good nutrition but may need some reminders or assistance to achieve this. Ancient ones may find that it is easier to "heat and eat" processed or prepared foods, but these are often high in salt and fat and low in fiber. In many cases, the diet of the elders is under the control of an organization such as Meals on Wheels, a national program that is geared toward improving nutrition for the nation's elderly, especially those with low income. This organization prepares and delivers nutritious meals to those unable to manage their shopping and cooking needs.

As families consider nutrition for elders, they need to consider all of these factors but also make choices that are based on the elder's real capability. It takes more time and effort to use fresh food and often it costs more (a struggle for elders on a tight budget). Fresh brussel sprouts may be nutritious—but only if the ancient one is able, willing, and/or has the assistance required to prepare them.

A healthy, balanced diet includes at least two and a half cups of (preferably fresh) fruit and vegetables every day; these foods are high in vitamins and fiber. While protein foods often include lean meat, fish, poultry, dairy, and eggs, it is quite healthy to have a plant-based diet with grains and legumes. Whole grain products have more fiber than "white" counterparts and should be selected whenever possible. Bread with even a little added whole grain is better than an all-white variety. Elders may find that some grains are easier to digest than others. For example, ancient ones may tolerate oats or barley better than whole wheat.

Many medical illnesses have a close relationship with food choice and habits. Certain foods worsen medical conditions; others put individuals at risk for further problems. These include

- sweets and simple sugars, which can cause high blood sugars;

- salt and high sodium in processed food, which can cause fluid retention, raise blood pressure, and increase tendency toward heart failure;

- high-fat foods, which can prompt a gallbladder problem and can raise cholesterol levels in blood, which is a risk factor for heart disease;

- high-acid foods, such as tomatoes and citrus, which can cause heartburn or reflux;

- high-potassium foods, such as bananas, potatoes, and tomatoes, which are not advised with kidney disease.

Diabetes is another complicated (and common condition) that affects diet. In many cases, food is both the cause and the treatment. The most common form of diabetes is adult onset, which is often a result of poor eating habits and obesity. In diabetes, the normal ways that the body controls blood sugar no longer work well. The result is elevated blood sugars, which over time cause trouble in almost all areas of the body. Diabetes is a risk factor for heart disease, stroke, kidney disease, circulation, and nerve problems. The timing and content of meals must be considered in relationship to medication and activity.

Dietary recommendations for the management of diabetes has shifted almost 360 degrees in the last fifty years. Currently the recommendations involve maintaining an ideal weight, avoiding concentrated sweets and simple carbohydrates, taking care not to skip meals, and eating healthy snacks. A consultation with a dietitian or diabetic education specialist is a very good idea. Medication issues related to diabetes will be discussed in Chapter 6.

Anyone who is on medication to lower blood sugar due to diabetes is at risk for problematic low blood sugar, which is called *hypoglycemia*. This is an unpleasant constellation of symptoms, including sweating, shaking, confusion, blurry vision, and—in the elderly—falls. This is an issue of trying to balance the medication with calories consumed. Care must be taken to not skip meals and always have a quick food source handy, such as candy, raisins, juice, or milk.

An elder can also end up with multiple medical conditions, each with its own set of dietary restrictions. For example, a diabetic with heart disease, kidney failure, and high cholesterol may be put on a low-carbohydrate, low-protein, low-salt, low-fat diet. Someone in this situation would be encouraged to avoid processed food and desserts and instead eat whole grains; vegetables (not potatoes or tomatoes), particularly green ones; minimal meat (especially avoiding red meat); and fish and chicken with no skin (baked, not fried).

The conflicting advice on restrictions can cause a lot of confusion. As noted, these restrictions are even more problematic if there are financial constraints, if meals are provided by an outside source (e.g., Meals on Wheels), or if there is a reliance on packaged convenience foods.

For a person with complex dietary needs, it's well worth the time to spend a few visits with a dietitian. Instead of just providing a list of what foods to avoid, a dietitian will provide lists of foods *to* eat and perhaps give tips on how to easily prepare them.

Of course, many chronic conditions have come about because of lifelong eating habits, so these habits may be the hardest to change. If a dietary regime is too complicated or unappealing, the elderly person will likely not follow it. In such cases, the suggestion of following a restrictive diet may actually result in malnutrition and undesirable weight loss. In some cases, it may be necessary to shift goals and conclude that for certain elders, the best food is the food that will be eaten.

Struggles with Eating

Aging creates physical problems that can interfere with eating and nutrition. Decreased sense of taste and smell can ruin an appetite. Dry mouth with diminished amounts of saliva points to the beginning of a slower digestive system. Oftentimes the end result is constipation, which can further decrease appetite. Here is one of the many "chicken and egg" situations. Reduced dietary intake contributes to reduced energy and strength. This will often result in less physical activity, which then worsens many other aspects of health, including appetite and life in general. All of these issues should be discussed with a doctor.

Tooth loss and other dental issues are common in the elderly and can result in nutritional problems. Dentures and partial plates are common and often have their own set of problems. Ancient ones must care for these devices daily, which can be a challenge. If eating is painful or just not fun any longer, then people stop eating. The problems with tooth loss and dentures can also cause self-consciousness, leading to social isolation. If this is occurring, a phone call or trip to the dentist may be in order.

The actual process of eating can also present challenges. Visual impairment, poor grip, or tremors can make it hard for ancient ones to get the food from the plate to their mouth. Strategies to minimize the effect of these problems include using plates with built-up edges, weighted utensils or those with special handles, and plates and placemats in contrasting colors to accommodate poor vision. Sometimes changes to things like finger foods or soup in a mug can improve overall intake, depending on what the problem is. Occupational therapy can also address problems of self-feeding.

Swallowing is another problem that relates to food intake and nutrition. The general population gives very little thought to this process, but it causes a lot of problems in the very old. A speech therapist is needed for this group of problems, which are discussed more fully later. (See the dysphasia diet in Chapter 7.) Basically, it's helpful to modify food and fluid textures to make the necessary process of swallowing easier.

Elders may also experience numerous symptoms related to the digestive system, and things can go wrong anywhere along the way. The gastrointestinal tract or GI system starts at the mouth and follows the food all the way out. These following symptoms are common:

- lack of appetite;

- nausea and vomiting;

- heartburn and indigestion;

- stomachache and cramps;

- bowel irregularity.

Some of these problems can occur suddenly and represent an acute event, but often they are gradual and creep up slowly, or they are intermittent and come and go. These symptoms may be caused by problems with food tolerance, GI pathology (disorders of the organs), medication side effects, and even stress. It is important to note any pattern of symptoms, such as

- timing of symptom related to food or medicine intake;

- activity or positioning, such as symptoms are worse when lying down;

- the presence of associated symptoms, such as pain or shortness of breath;

- things that make symptoms better; and

- things that make symptoms worse.

These observations can help direct healthcare providers to the root of the problem.

Mary's story illustrates a few of the food-based issues that can arise as elders age and their lifestyles change. In Mary's case, there was no specific event that triggered her decline, and up to this point, her family felt she was "getting by fine."

Mary

Mary is an eighty-seven-year-old widow who tripped on a rug and fell at the family home in which she had lived for forty-six years. In spite of having no broken bones, she was still badly bruised. She was admitted for physical rehab, did well, and soon returned home. In general, her health was pretty good. Although her three daughters lived out of state, her two sons lived nearby. They took her to lunch and helped her run errands such as grocery shopping once a week.

Prior to her husband's death, Mary had weighed 125 pounds. However, during the past three years, her weight had dropped to 92. She reported that she did not have much of an appetite anymore, and she wasn't getting much exercise. A medical evaluation attempted to find an explanation for her weight loss, but nothing was identified. She was neither depressed nor demented.

As part of the follow-up to Mary's rehabilitation, she received treatments at home. During one of these visits, her routine was observed by an occupational therapist, who asked Mary to simulate preparing a meal. Throughout the simulation, Mary continually looked at the big pots and pans she still had on hand from younger days when she needed to feed a crowd. She ate her meal at the counter because old catalogs, newspapers, and junk mail had claimed her dining table. The clutter was creating an unappealing atmosphere for meals and a less than safe environment. To the therapist, it was apparent that Mary was disinclined to prepare food for herself, finding it to be too much of a bother.

Several recommendations were made. The kitchen was reorganized to move the daily use items for easy reach and to remove appliances and items that were used only on rare occasions. Mary hadn't kept up with trash removal and recycling, so an improved plan for tidying up was created. Her son brought in a few new, smaller pots that made it easier to cook for one, and the sons set up a small table as a pleasant spot for a solitary meal. They took up the rag rug floor runner as a safety precaution.

Finally, a social worker connected Mary with the local senior service organization. Here she was able to get help with shopping and housework to fill in the gaps between her own functioning and the things her family could do for her. The sons were happy to be given directions on how to foster their mother's independence, safety, and well-being—and Mary was willing to accept the changes that supported her continued independence.

Even with the best of care and a comprehensive tightly woven safety net, decline at some point becomes inevitable. The next few chapters discuss how to access the healthcare system, some of the frequent issues surrounding common medical problems, and some of the difficulties with medical evaluations and treatments for people of advanced age.

Chapter Five

Accessing the Healthcare System

Accessing the healthcare system on the behalf of an elderly family member can be done in one of three ways:

- planned out with thought and intention;
- intermittent and half-involved; and more commonly
- in the midst of a crisis.

Often the ancient ones who now need medical care were previously independent, discussing care with only their healthcare providers, and relating select information to family. However, issues may suddenly rise to the surface, particularly when friends or family members start to worry that there may not be a clear understanding between the patients and providers. Then there reaches a point when the primary care provider gets the "I'm worried about Mom call." The family members either want information from the medical provider or else they are providing information to make sure the particular symptom or other problem is known and addressed.

As our ancient ones seek and require treatment, family members may want to be included in the process. Ideally, a family member can accompany the elder to some, or all, medical appointments, or at least when there is a particular concern. If this is not possible, then with the patient's consent, dialogues with healthcare providers must take place over the phone, which may be adequate but is not the optimum situation.

Health Insurance Portability and Accountability Act (HIPAA) and Communication

It is important to note that a federal regulation called HIPAA (Health Insurance Portability and Accountability Act), which protects the individual's right of privacy, affects this communication. This may not be a problem if the elder consents to the sharing of information between the healthcare team and the family. However, healthcare providers *must receive explicit permission from the patient (or their healthcare proxy if that has been activated) to allow them to talk to anyone else about the patient's condition.* This permission can be simply noted in the medical record with no special forms required. Oftentimes, one family member is the contact person and information can go to other interested parties through that person. Keep in mind there is no special permission needed for the healthcare provider to listen to any information from concerned family or friends.

If the patient hasn't granted this permission, either on purpose or as an oversight, the dialogue will be limited. Ancient ones may choose to keep their own healthcare issues to themselves for a variety of reasons. For instance, they may want to prevent their families from worrying, or they could be trying to cover up a medical or functional decline. They may resist interference from well-intentioned family members because they fear limitations on their activities or intrusions upon their current style of life.

With this in mind, it can be quite essential for the ancient ones to have a caregiver, family member, or advocate to accompany them to medical appointments and, as needed, make phone calls on their behalf. Communication difficulties are common during medical evaluations and can create problems when healthcare providers don't understand the elder's question or description and address a different issue instead. If this continues to occur, it may be time to try a different health care provider instead.

In other cases, healthcare providers may mislabel patients as confused when in fact they are actually well oriented but merely hard of hearing. In fact, even elders with good hearing may have difficulty speaking during an appointment. Dry mouth, dental loss, soft voice, or garbled speech can impair the ability for expression. Native accents may become more pronounced in stressful situations and as age progresses, and often ancient ones begin to revert to their original language. Communication impairment can blur the distinctions between dementia, depression, mental clarity, and comprehension. Sadly, elderly people with these communication impairments often aren't fully included from participating in the decision-making process.

Needless to say, all of these situations can make assessments difficult. As an advocate for the elderly patient, it is important to make sure that the ancient one can hear and understand *and* is heard and understood.

A crisis situation further amplifies these issues. When family members are brought into the scene in response to an urgent medical event, they may find themselves in an official or impromptu family meeting to discuss the problem. If there is a high level of urgency, as occurs when a medical crisis brings the family together in the hospital's emergency department, then the family may have a brief discussion about the patient's desires related to life support (see Chapter 6).

The best time to discuss all of these situations—who will take Dad to the doctor, who is authorized to speak with Dad's healthcare team, and what end-of-life instructions are in place—is *before* an illness sets things in motion. If your family has not come to agreement on these issues, now would be a great time to do so.

The Various Roles of the Healthcare Support Team

The cast of characters involved in healthcare and services is long and can be confusing. There are many layers of personnel, all with differing educational preparation, qualifications, experience, and role in the care of the ancient ones.[2]

PRIMARY CARE PHYSICIANS

The trends in insurance management support the idea of having a gatekeeper of all medical care. In the present format, the top of the hierarchy is the *primary care physician* (*PCP*).[3] This is a professional who is either a medical doctor (MD) or doctor of osteopathy (DO), and specializes in either internal medicine or family practice (or pediatrics when dealing with children). This doctor was formerly called a *general practitioner* or a *family doctor*.

The term *PCP* can also refer to the *primary care provider* if this person is not a physician. A nurse practitioner (NP) and physician assistant (PA) fill this role in many settings; those professionals are described in their own section of this chapter.

PHYSICIAN SPECIALISTS

Physician specialists are doctors whose practices are limited to one area of concern. Examples include cardiologists or heart specialists; orthopedists, who specialize in bones and joints; pulmonologists, who are lung and breathing specialists; and neurologists for those with neurological conditions such as Parkinson's Disease—to name a very few. Specialists are meant to focus on their narrow area of concern and are not intended to focus on the "big picture" of how the person's whole health is going. These highly skilled practitioners have a great deal

---

[2] While the following discussion of healthcare providers details the common traditional roles, this is not meant to exclude alternative health practitioners, such as chiropractors, acupuncturists, herbalists, massage therapists, and energy workers. This group is in evolution, and their credibility is increasing as their respective fields demonstrate merit. I believe there is a huge amount of untapped potential for these modalities in the care of our elders, and over time we will see increased utilization with improved outcomes, with more coverage for these services included in insurance plans.

[3] There are some who think that it is the insurance companies that really are at the top of the medical hierarchy, followed closely by the drug companies. However, that debate goes beyond the scope of this discussion.

of expertise, particularly with regard to the diagnosis and treatment of problems within their fields. They may be consulted only a time or two to establish a treatment plan, or they may be consulted on an ongoing basis to follow up with care.

Ideally, when PCPs refer elders to known specialists, the ancient ones will receive appropriate high-quality care. Seeing a specialist can help patients and their families sort out the wide range of healthcare options available in our complicated world. Both PCPs and specialists are graduates from medical school, are board certified in their respective fields, and are licensed by the state in which they practice. They have completed a credentialing process for all of the institutions, hospitals, and other facilities in which they practice.

With this in mind, when patients are seeing both a PCP and a specialist, it is in the patient's best interest for the PCP and the specialist to have a dialogue in all situations when ongoing follow-up care is needed. This is especially important when the healthcare providers are on different computer systems and may not have immediate access to each other's notes. In these situations, it's also essential to ensure that services and medications aren't duplicated or conflicting.

NURSES

Nursing is a field made up of individuals with a wide range of educational preparation. *Licensed practical nurses* or *LPNs* (*LVNs* for *licensed vocational nurses* in some states) are educated in a one- or two-year program, usually in a vocational school setting. The education is practicality oriented, rather than academically based, and they receive a diploma or certification for completion of the program.

In contrast, the education of a *registered nurse* or *RN* may have taken place at a community college, resulting in an associate degree; at a four-year college, resulting in a bachelor's degree; or (formerly) at a hospital-based program, resulting in a diploma in nursing. This diploma program was the most common form of education years ago, but now it's been all but phased out, with a trend toward college-based programs.

RNs and LPNs have passed a qualifying exam for their level of practice, are licensed by a state board, and are prepared to work in a multitude of healthcare settings.

Registered nurses can also become certified in a given specialty by studying and passing a standardized examination. The specialties range from prenatal to geriatrics and from intensive care in highly technical environments to community-based home care. Overall, there

Primary Nursing and Team Nursing

Primary nursing is done in a setting where one nurse at a time is responsible for all the patient's needs, from monitoring and meds to personal care. This is done in hospitals much more than in rehab or long-term care settings, where team nursing is the norm.

In *team nursing* there are usually higher nurse-to-patient ratios, and the tasks of care are divided among several caregivers. One of the more visible and accessible players is the *charge nurse*. The nurse in this role communicates with physicians and other disciplines to report problems, receive orders about medication and treatments, and organize the implementation of these orders. The charge nurse then delegates to *staff nurses*, who are responsible for assessing patients, administering medications, and performing treatments, such as wound care. The nurses also are responsible for the supervision and delegation of personal care provided by the nurse's aides.

are more opportunities for advancement for RNs than for LPNs, including administration, education, public health, case management, and private business. However, LPNs and RNs—particularly in rehabs and long-term care settings—often work side by side with little or no difference in job description or job performance.

Nurses work in all sorts of settings: hospitals, rehabs, nursing homes, community health centers, home care agencies, and schools. Any inpatient healthcare setting is likely to have a director of nursing, an assistant director of nursing, nursing supervisors, and/or nurse managers. These upper-level nurses have varying degrees of visibility and can be called upon for difficult situations.

The structures of nursing care are usually based upon the specific needs of the patients and the available staff. Families, patients, and caregivers should ask someone at the individual facility to explain the care system, whom to talk to on a daily basis, and where to get the big picture. For instance, in some situations, *nurse case managers* monitor the situation, try to facilitate patient care, and communicate with families as the patient progresses through the system. That progression may occur within an isolated hospitalization or through a complicated illness in and out of multiple healthcare institutions. Nurse case managers may work for inpatient facilities, physician group practices, or in the managed care system.

ADVANCED PRACTICE REGISTERED NURSES

Advanced practice registered nurse (ARNP) is the general term that includes nurse practitioners, certified nurse midwives, nurse anesthetists, and clinical nurse specialists. Nurses with this specialized education are master-level prepared nurses with state licenses and national certification in a specialty. Nurse practitioners work in settings such as family practice, adult medicine, geriatrics, or pediatrics. Midwives work in women's health and obstetrics. Anesthetists work in surgical settings, and clinical nurse specialists often work in psychiatry. They are considered to be "mid-level" practitioners, situated between the traditional physician and nursing roles. Advance practice nurses assume many of the roles previously performed by physicians, including the diagnosis and treatment of common problems, both acute and chronic. Plans are in place to elevate the educational preparation of nurse practitioners to the doctorate level.

PHYSICIAN ASSISTANTS

Physician assistants represent another type of "mid-level practitioner." Like nurse practitioners, they perform duties formerly handled by doctors, including routine medicine, and some also assist with surgery and specialized procedures. Initially, physician assistants were used and developed by the military, but training is now done in academic settings. They also work in collaboration with physicians to provide high-quality care for patients in a variety of settings, ranging from office-based practices to specialties to the operating room.

PHYSICAL, OCCUPATIONAL, AND SPEECH THERAPISTS

Rehabilitation staff play an important part in the care of the elderly. There are roles for these therapists in acute care hospitals, in rehabilitation hospitals, in nursing homes, and in home care. Physical, occupational, and speech therapies are different disciplines that work closely together in geriatric settings. These therapists have been educated at the bachelor's, master's, or doctorate level, although the graduate level of training is favored and may soon be the required degree.

Physical therapists focus on strengthening exercises, endurance, and stability of ambulation. They also may have specialized training in pain management, using therapeutic modalities such as heat, ice, ultrasound, and electrical stimulation.

Occupational therapists work on issues of functionality, such as bathing, dressing, and moving through tasks of daily living with safety and care.

Both physical and occupational therapists may use assistants as part of a team-based approach toward progress. These *therapy assistants* have associates degrees and work under the supervision of the registered therapist. Typically, the registered therapist performs the evaluations of the patient and then sets up a treatment plan with individualized goals, while the assistant actually implements that plan. The plans are re-evaluated by the team on regular intervals as progress is made or not made.

Speech therapists assess and treat cognition, speaking, and alternate forms of communication, such as keyboards. The therapist also can evaluate mental status, help identify the areas of difficulties in thought process, and arrive at strategies to compensate for problems. Swallowing and mastication are other areas of concern for speech therapists. They are the ones who make recommendations regarding dietary textures.

CERTIFIED NURSING ASSISTANTS

Certified nursing assistants or *CNAs* (also called *orderlies, health techs, nursing aides,* or *home health aides*) are individuals trained, in four to six weeks, to perform a variety of basic tasks related to personal care, bathing, dressing, and toileting. At times, depending on the setting, CNAs can perform more advanced tasks, such as wound care or even med administration, under the supervision of a nurse. The training period is brief, so the degree of competence is often dependent on aptitude and disposition. CNAs work in hospitals, rehabs, nursing homes, and in-home care. Nursing aides make up the backbone of the long-term care in institutions and in the community. They provide valuable information about the small details of daily life and can, if observant, provide early warnings of serious changes.

HOMEMAKERS

Homemakers are people who provide housekeeping and do chores such as cleaning, laundry, shopping, and (sometimes) cooking, but they generally do not perform any degree of personal care. Families and patients can hire these workers independently, or they can come through a home care program that orchestrates the services to meet particular individual needs. Elderly patients sometimes hire *companions* to provide company, supervision, and minor assistance, though not for personal care. In a hospital situation, restless or confused patients may need the extra attention of a companion (who is then called a *sitter*) for one-on-one supervision to ensure safety.

MENTAL HEALTHCARE PROFESSIONALS

Mental health is a big area in the care of elders. (See Chapter 9.) This field involves numerous providers, briefly summarized here.

- *Psychiatrists* are medical doctors with specialization in the treatment of mental and behavioral illness. They are the experts in the drug therapies for these problems.

- *Advance practice nurses* also advise and prescribe medications in mental health situations.

- *Psychologists, therapists,* and *counselors* have masters or doctorate level preparation in psychology, social work, or mental health. They are involved in the talk therapy part of mental healthcare.

- *Social workers* are instrumental in setting up home services for elders who are being discharged from a healthcare institution. They are the most familiar with the community resources and how to utilize them. They are employed by hospitals, rehabilitation centers, nursing homes, and a variety of community-based organizations.

* * *

From physicians to nursing aides, all healthcare providers are required to undergo ongoing continuing education to keep up with the ever-changing world of healthcare.

The knowledge of the role each of these team members plays will help the patient advocate connect with the appropriate member for any of the numerous issues that are bound to come up during the illness and recovery of an elderly patient. It may be very useful to start and maintain a caregiver's journal to help keep the players straight. In the next chapter, we'll discuss steps for evaluation when elders show symptoms of physical or mental distress.

Chapter Six

Trouble Brewing

In general, we measure our own good health by the subjective feeling of well-being, an absence of unpleasant symptoms, and our ability to perform our required daily activities. When our health status declines and new symptoms or a rapid progression of symptoms develop, as alert adults we hope to recognize situations that require medical attention. When we have slower, vague changes, we discuss them with our healthcare providers at routine medical visits. And if problems progress over a few days, such as respiratory complaints, then we schedule an extra office visit to check out the symptoms.

With that in mind, it can be harder to measure the good health of the ancient ones, particularly if they are vague or not forthcoming about their symptoms. As the ancient ones' health fluctuates, it is important for the patients or their advocate to be able to identify, quantify, and communicate these changes to healthcare providers in order to get the proper attention. Having a working vocabulary of these terms and issues empowers patients and their families to discuss them in a meaningful way. The following strategies will help you recognize the deviations from the baseline and the trends in the health of the very old as they impact daily life, as well as how to communicate with various members of the healthcare team, and what to expect from these encounters.

Assessing the Elder's Physical and Mental Condition

Increased concern for the well-being of a frail elder begins when observers realize something is amiss. Something is not quite right, and it's important to identify and quantify how serious it is. This section describes a series of things to consider when planning an encounter with a medical professional. The family's observations and ability to clearly and concisely report them provides invaluable information for the healthcare team to make a diagnosis and come up with an appropriate plan.

Time is often short in medical visits, and these older people are generally slow moving; some also have communication impairments. Whenever possible, collect the following pieces of background information before interacting with medical professionals. It's also important to provide specific medical information in terms of reporting medication compliance, reactions to medications, as well as the timing of symptoms related to medications. Having all of this information readily available for the medical appointment will allow for improved use of time for discussion and actual problem solving.

WHAT IS THE TIMEFRAME OF THE CHANGES?

In most cases healthcare providers will ask caregivers to provide a clear chronological review. To begin, start by considering the basics. What is the timeframe of the changes? The problems that evolve over days or weeks are a different order of business than the problems that develop over minutes or hours. Generally, serious problems that are worsening over minutes or hours are more appropriate for the emergency department, whereas problems worsening over days may be seen in the office today or tomorrow. Problems that come and go, or are not particularly troublesome, can wait a few days for a convenient appointment. It is also useful to keep a running list of concerns that can be brought to regularly scheduled appointments.

WHAT IS THE ELDER'S OVERALL APPEARANCE?

Caregivers can obtain a good deal of information by observing the elderly person's general appearance.

- Is there any visible distress?

- Does the elder seem alert, calm, or agitated?

- Is there evidence of discomfort or pain?

- Is there a noticeable difference from the elder's usual appearance?

Grooming and appropriateness of clothing can provide clues about physical and cognitive functioning. Any change in the interest in or ability for self-care is a serious symptom. Confusion can sometimes lead to some rather unique outfits, without regard to the circumstances or weather. For example, I have seen a patient wear pantyhose over her slacks, upside-down shirts (no small feat!), and heavy coats in the heat of the summer.

HOW'S THE BREATHING?

Caregivers who know what to look for can determine the patient's quality of respiration. Normal breathing should be effortless. Shortness of breath (SOB) is the most common symptom of breathing troubles; this describes the feeling of just not getting enough air. This may be subjective, with no visible changes apparent to the observer. Other times there may be very objective physical findings.

Activity will often change the quality of respiration. The person may be using extra muscles in the chest and shoulders to move the air in and out. This is labored breathing. It is important to note a change in breathing in response to activity, both in terms of how much activity prompts breathlessness, and the time needed to recover to normal breathing. If a person cannot speak due to shortness of breath, this is a case of extreme labored breathing.

Healthcare providers evaluate breath and breathing by several methods. The most basic is respiratory rate, which is the number of complete respiratory cycles (one inhalation and one exhalation) in a minute. This is determined by counting the breath as the chest rises and falls with each cycle. The normal respiratory rate is approximately 18 to 22 respirations a minute. The respiratory rate is normally increased in response to exertion but should promptly return to baseline. An infection, such as pneumonia, COPD (chronic lung disease) exacerbation, or even anxiety can increase a person's respiratory rate, which can be an early warning sign of problems ahead. Using the ear alone or a stethoscope, providers may also hear the person make extra sounds associated with respirations.

Cough is a common occurrence that can hamper breathing, and caregivers should look for severity, frequency, and whether the timing is related to activity, or food or fluid intake. There are several kinds of cough. A productive cough will produce sputum or phlegm. The color, amount, and consistency of sputum are unpleasant to observe but important enough to check out, even if the caregiver has to spy on the inner sides of used tissues. Colored sputum can often indicate a more severe problem.

A nonproductive or dry cough may be frequent and bothersome. A wheeze is the whistling sound of air being trapped in the air passages. A caregiver may notice a moist rattling sound or gurgling at different times of the day. Try to notice the timing and circumstances of these events.

Auscultation refers to using a stethoscope to listen to the breath or other sounds. This allows for amplification of physiological sounds. A skilled listener can determine the quality of air movement, wheezing, and accumulation of fluids that is present in pneumonia and congestive heart failure.

HOW'S THE HEART PUMPING?

A well-working heart gives a body the look of aliveness. A pallor that is ashen or a dusky color is often a sign of heart problems. As the heart beats, it is pumping the blood throughout the body. Checking the pulse—either by feeling the beats at the wrist or neck or listening with a stethoscope to the chest—monitors movement of the blood. Both the rate (number of beats per minute) and rhythm (the regularity) are evaluated this way.

Blood pressure is another sign of cardiovascular functioning, and this is checked easily at home with automatic or manual devices. While blood pressure readings are taken at many healthcare encounters, it is useful for those with blood pressure problems to take independent readings (and record them) to see the fluctuations over the course of time.

HOW'S THE MENTAL STATUS?

This is a complex assessment that reflects the interplay of many factors:

- level of alertness or wakefulness;

- cognitive or thinking status; and

- mood.

Mental status and thinking are complex processes that affect all aspects of a person's well-being. The first assessment can be centered around the different "levels of consciousness," which refer to the ability of the body to have awareness of the world around themselves. It describes how awake the elder is. Here are the different levels of consciousness, from the largest to least decline.

- *Coma* and *semi-coma* are low on the continuum of responsiveness; people in a semi-coma require vigorous touch to elicit any response, while people in a coma give no response to activities, such as personal care or repositioning. This is common at end of life.

- A *stuporous* person needs more stimulation than a loud voice—perhaps a shake to rouse—and may easily drift off; if this level of consciousness diminishes, more stimulation is required to elicit a response.

- *Lethargic* is the next status; the person is sleepy and, though able to respond to a variety of stimuli, will give responses that are a little fuzzy and possibly delayed.

- *Alert* is the highest level; the brain is awake and able to respond to any of a variety of stimuli, including things that can be seen, heard, or felt. This is the way most people are when awake. A fully alert person is able to respond to verbal and nonverbal communication, as well as other aspects of the environment.

This assessment is seemingly crude, but it serves as a very important indicator of the degree of health or illness, and caregivers can easily judge and communicate these factors to healthcare providers.

The next factor that is used to access cognition is orientation. This reflects the elders' awareness of their place in the world. Fully functional people are oriented to

- person (they know their name and the names of other familiar people);
- place (they know where they are, where they have been, or where they "belong");
- time (they know the day of the week, the date, the year, the season); and
- circumstance (they know about their health situation, their living arrangements, and recent events).

The degree of orientation may change slowly over time or may vary greatly over the course of a day. For instance, *sundowning* is a term used for the predictable worsening of mental status that occurs in the afternoon or evening in demented persons (just as an infant is prone to colic during these times). Any change in level of orientation from baseline is important as it may reflect a change in medical status or help define a pattern of behavior.

Other components of cognition are

- insight (the elders' ability to comprehend complex situations or recognize their own current situation);
- judgment (their ability to make decisions or plan a course of action to an unexpected event); and
- short-, and long-term memory (e.g., remembering what they ate for breakfast versus remembering events from long ago).

Mood or *affect* is an assessment made with regard to personality manifestation. The mood may be depressed, anxious, agitated, or calm and cooperative. Mood may remain relatively constant or change through the day. Caregivers should identify trends in mood that limit function, such as depression, anxiety, or agitation, as these are problems that healthcare providers should treat. Note that not all treatment needs to be pharmacological. Many behavioral interventions can be effective. (These will be discussed further in Chapter 9.) The earlier the caregivers or patients note the problems, the easier it may be for the healthcare providers to make improvements.

Behavior is the manifestation of mood. Changes in behavior can come suddenly or shift slowly over days or weeks. There are times when elders are just "not acting themselves," and that is reason enough to seek medical attention.

HOW WELL IS THE PERSON MOVING ABOUT?

Mobility and coordination are important things to notice, and changes are common.

- Do all body parts (arms and legs, hands and feet) move spontaneously?

- Has there been a fall? How did it occur (tripping, fainting, or prompted by dizziness)?

- Are there abnormal movements such as tremors, twitching, or shaking?

- Is there a change in strength, such as trouble getting out of the chair or walking, or a decrease in endurance?

- Is there a limp, unsteadiness, or a shuffling gait?

Changes in mobility may occur for a variety of reasons, and may come on suddenly or progress over days to weeks. Generalized weakness or an unsteady pattern of walking may be from simple fatigue or an early indicator of impending illness. Rest and monitoring for progression is reasonable. These things can be discussed in a planned office visit.

Problems that come on suddenly and reflect a major change, such as loss of function of a limb, need emergency evaluation.

Any decline in mobility in frail or marginally functioning elders may increase their need for assistance and the feasibility of living at home without help may suddenly change.

HAS THERE BEEN A CHANGE IN EATING HABITS?

Appetite and fluid intake are important factors to observe. Note whether changes in intake are sudden or developing over days or weeks. In emergency situations it may be important to note when and what was the last food or fluid consumed.

HAS THERE BEEN A CHANGE IN BATHROOM HABITS?

Problems with elimination are big concerns for the elderly, but they may find it difficult to discuss these issues. Alternatively, some ancient ones may be more interested in this topic than any other. Isolated changes and symptoms, as well as changing patterns, are important to note, including incontinence or accidents. These topics are extensively addressed in Chapter 7.

ARE THERE ANY SKIN CHANGES?

The skin is the body's largest organ, and it reflects what's going on in the body as a whole. Overall color is important.

- Pallor can reflect anemia.

- Grey or bluish skin often indicates a circulatory problem.

- Flushed red skin can indicate fever.

- Yellow or orange skin can indicate liver disease.

Skin should be warm and dry, and when the skin on the back of the hand is pinched, it should return to place. Aside from sweat, fluids should never leak from the skin.

Here are more symptoms to look for on the skin.

- Areas of increased warmth, redness, or swelling can indicate infection or inflammation.

- Dry, cracked lips, or sunken, dry eyes are signs of dehydration.

- Sweating can be tied with a fever, low blood sugar, or even a heart attack.

- Bumps, bruises, burns, and cuts can show up with no explanation; these provide suspicion for unreported falls, smoking, or cooking mishaps.

- Rashes, which may indicate a medical condition, medication reaction, or personal care problems, may show up anywhere, but skin folds, hands, and legs are common rash locations.

These concerns are in addition to the usual ubiquitous skin oddities of the very old. *Raised, warty, rough, scaly,* and *crusty* are just some of the descriptions of skin lesions that commonly develop. Many are cosmetic issues or just bothersome, but some indicate cancer. Any skin lesion that changes with increasing size, bleeds, or is otherwise worrisome should be brought to the attention of a medical provider.

* * *

The information gleaned by all of these assessments will help caregivers identify problems and communicate them to the healthcare provider.

Medical Evaluations

A medical evaluation usually follows these general steps:

1. Identification of complaint, symptoms, and signs

2. Evaluation

3. Diagnosis

4. Treatment

This is actually a complicated process that is much like a puzzle with many pieces. The following section is meant to help demystify the experience, including the jargon used by medical professionals.

STEP 1: IDENTIFICATION OF COMPLAINT, SYMPTOMS, AND SIGNS

The medical practitioner first considers the patient's complaint, symptoms, and signs. The *chief complaint* is the phrase that describes why the elder is seeking medical attention. This may be a vague complaint, such as "Mom is not quite right," or specific, as in cough or back pain.

The *symptoms* are a subjective perception of the elder's body, related to illness or discomfort. It includes the details about severity, timing, associated symptoms, and what makes the symptoms better or worse. This information is called the "history" of the problem and may be provided by patients, their family, or caregivers.

Symptoms in an elderly person are often vague. *Generalized* or *constitutional symptoms* are common symptoms, such as weakness, dizziness, fatigue, and mental status change. There may not be an obvious relationship between the symptom and the source of the problem. These vague symptoms can involve the beginning of a new problem, an exacerbation of a chronic problem, a side effect of many medications, or a combination of all of these.

Focal or *localized symptoms* relate to the specific problem area, such as joint pain in an injured joint. The problem in this case is usually related to the area of complaint (for instance, knee pain usually relates to a problem with the knee).

A *sign* is an objective finding identified through the hands-on examination or the "physical" part of the medical encounter. This includes vital signs (temperature, pulse, respiratory rate, and blood pressure), or any observable findings like a cough and wheeze, lumps and bumps, redness and swelling, or change in mental status.

STEP 2: EVALUATION

The problem or problems will then be evaluated or "worked up." The *differential diagnosis* is a thinking process, by the healthcare provider, considering all of the possible causes for the problem. Medical tests may be ordered that will add important information or data to help complete the picture.

One thing that doctors will be trying to determine is whether the signs are indicative of an acute or a chronic illness. Let's take a brief moment to review what these terms mean.

Acute and Chronic Illness

Illness is divided into two main categories: *acute* and *chronic*. An *acute illness* develops fairly suddenly, has a short duration, and comes with the expectation that it will resolve with treatment or time. Examples of this type of illness are

- viral infections, such as colds and flu;

- bronchitis and pneumonia;

- urinary tract infections;

- acute arthritis and gout;

- stomach or bowel problems such as nausea, vomiting, or diarrhea.

These acute problems in a younger population are usually simple and straightforward. However, the ancient ones rarely have simple or straightforward situations of *any* kind, including medical. Instead, these new acute conditions are likely to add another layer of concern onto an already compromised elder.

Acute or sudden illness is often superimposed upon chronic illness. This can result in a formerly well-controlled situation going to pieces due to an infection or other new problem, such as a fall that necessitates pain medications, which then cause unpleasant side effects. Changes in condition are subtle and can result in symptoms that may not be so obvious to the untrained person. Elders who are normally well oriented may become confused, or their mental status may begin to deteriorate. This may develop quickly or become apparent in a few days or even weeks later.

For instance, people with well-controlled diabetes can suddenly experience very high blood sugar when an acute infection is brewing, regardless of the source of infection. Prompt medical treatment for acute conditions can help to decrease the duration and intensity of these problems.

Chronic illnesses are much more involved. These are often lifelong conditions or diseases that may change in severity but do not really go away. Some chronic conditions, such as high blood pressure, have no symptoms, while others, such as arthritis, can impact every step of life. As noted, chronic conditions also make every acute illness more serious. Examples of chronic illness are

- heart disease, congestive heart failure, coronary artery disease, atrial fibrillation;
- respiratory disease, COPD, asthma, emphysema;
- diabetes (all kinds);
- arthritis (rheumatoid, osteoarthritis, and gout);
- cancers (all kinds);
- psychiatric or mental illness, depression, anxiety;
- dementia, including Alzheimer's disease.

Due to improved healthcare, a higher standard of living, and better support systems, many people are now living with chronic illnesses that were once considered fatal. In fact, many people have a constellation of chronic illnesses that are in need of careful and skilled medical management involving lifestyle adaptation and medication. These conditions are ongoing in nature, often progressive, and have periods of quiescence and exacerbations. In other words, these are problems that come and go with flare-ups and improvement, but generally they do get worse over time.

Managing multiple medical conditions is a challenging and complex task. Often the treatment of one condition negatively impacts the course of another. It is the interaction between these discreet conditions and all of their associated medications that make the overall management so complicated. In some cases, the effects of the medications are predictable. For instance, constipation from pain medicines can be anticipated and avoided with laxatives. In these instances, the benefits of treating a medical problem can outweigh the manageable side effects. Careful monitoring of symptoms and lab tests will help to minimize these risks.

Unfortunately, there are times when someone is truly "stuck between a rock and a hard place" in the treatment of one or more problems with the goal of doing the least harm for the greatest amount of good. In these cases, when decisions for treatment need to be made, it's important for caregivers to ask healthcare providers to review the various approaches and the likely scenarios that will occur as a result of each possible treatment.

STEP 3: DIAGNOSIS

During this diagnostic phase, the healthcare provider attempts to exclude or "rule out" many possibilities as the evidence develops. A final diagnosis will be made through the integration of information obtained from the history, the physical exam, and diagnostic studies, which are the focus of this section.

Selecting the best (if any) tests for elderly patients can be a complicated matter. In very basic terms, some tests show blood or body composition; others reveal structure or function of body parts. This information provides pieces of the puzzle of a particular problem. Diagnostic testing can range from simple to complex.

Traditionally, doctors and patients have expected that tests should be ordered and undertaken until the specific problem is revealed. However, for those of very advanced age, it is wise to first consider the issues surrounding the tests and the practicalities of where the test must occur and how the patients will get there, as well as what will happen to them during the test. For instance, for elders with anxiety, fears about procedures can keep them awake for days in advance of the test. Long bumpy rides in cars or ambulances are exhausting and uncomfortable. It may be difficult for patients to get on and off the exam tables. Often, the procedures alone result in ordeals that can take days to get over.

It's also important to consider that all medical procedures require some level of cooperation. For example, some tests require a "prep." This may just involve fasting for several hours or it may require a complicated regime of liquids and laxatives and a complete bowel cleanse. This is no fun at any age, but it can be very debilitating for the elderly.

Cognitive decline, hearing loss, anxiety, and restlessness can limit the quality of any diagnostic testing. It can be impossible for some ancient ones to hold completely still and then move in a specific way on command. Lack of cooperation for blood draws can increase the discomfort of the activity, and it can make imaging studies produce a result that is less than clear. If stillness for a procedure is required but unlikely, then some level of sedation may be needed. With all these potential problems, it is important to be sure the test is worth doing and the results will provide information that will have meaningful impact on the treatment plan.

The following section contains a brief description of common medical tests to help you make good decisions about diagnostic procedures.

Blood Tests

Blood tests can identify many problems about organ function and response to illness. These tests are done by a venipuncture, which involves threading a needle into a vein and withdrawing enough blood to fill one or more small tubes for analysis.

For most of the adult population, blood draws are usually a simple procedure. However, in the very old, nothing is simple. Veins are delicate, and it is much more difficult to obtain a sample. Sometimes several attempts are needed, each with its own poke, and each poke hurts. Patient cooperation is also required. Elders must hold their arm still; in the absence of that, as in dementia, the patient's arm needs restraining, making the whole process that much more difficult. Bruising of arms is common with repeated needlesticks, which is often done in hospitalized patients.

Urine Tests

Urine tests are commonly ordered for the elderly. The *urinalysis* provides immediate information about what is in the urine and the status of the patient. Among other things, it can indicate with some certainty the likelihood of infection.

The *culture and sensitivity* part of a urine test provides a further investigation, identifying the exact germ and what antibiotic will be useful. This second test takes two or three days to complete.

Fingersticks

Some simple tests can be performed independently with a drop of blood, which is usually obtained by a sharp prick to a fingertip during a procedure called a *fingerstick*. A lancet (a small pin-tipped poker) is used to obtain this drop of blood. In the case of diabetes, this drop of blood is put on a test strip, which is inserted into a little handheld machine called a *glucometer*. The glucometer provides a digital reading to indicate the blood sugar level. These machines also keep a log of the readings so users and their healthcare providers can review recent levels easily and identify trends. This is a cornerstone of diabetic management, and it provides information for medication dosing.

Mastering this skill requires the desire to do so, sufficiently nimble fingers, and adequate vision. Elders also need to comprehend when to do this and what to do about the results. This is often prohibitively difficult with ancient ones, so this frequently becomes a delegated task.

Urine Samples

A urine sample is needed when there is reason to suspect a urinary tract infection (UTI). However, if the urine specimen is improperly obtained, it may be contaminated, making the specimen of little value, which can then delay treatment. A "clean catch" urine is usually requested. However, this is not an easy project for an elderly person. The sample should be collected in a sterile specimen cup or, if the lab allows, a jar from the dishwasher. Before urinating, the area around the urethra must be cleaned. Next, the ancient one first pees in the toilet; then pees in the cup, collecting a midstream sample; and then finishes peeing in the toilet. Then the cup is closed and returned to the lab.

Another approach that can be used with ancient ones who are unable to follow directions, either because of physical or cognitive limitations, is a "straight catch" specimen. A nurse can easily obtain urine this way, and it can be a more reliable method to get the needed specimen. The external genitalia are thoroughly cleaned, a small tube is passed through the urethra, and the urine is collected into a specimen cup.

Imaging Studies

Imaging studies refer to things such as ultrasound, x-ray, CT, and MRI. These use different methods to get a "picture" of what is going on inside the body. Some of these tests need *contrast medium*, to help get a good image of body structure. This is either a drink that needs to be taken at a specific time or a dye that is injected into a vein; both may be needed. All of these have limitations, and each test has things it is able to do well and other things it does poorly. For complicated problems it may be necessary to have several tests done for a complete evaluation.

Plain x-rays, although generally quick and easy, are limited to identifying bone problems and some common lung problems. x-ray equipment is widely available and extended travel is not needed.

Both CT and MRI scans, depending on the specific machine, may require the patient to tolerate being in a closed space, which can be difficult for many very old people. MRIs are not quick and can take over an hour. They also have irregular loud banging, which can be upsetting for the patient.

All imaging studies need patient cooperation, as absolute stillness is required for the duration of the procedure. The aftereffects from these various imagining tests include discomfort due to travel or lying on the exam table, and constipation or diarrhea from the contrast drink.

Biopsies

Biopsies are a diagnostic study done on tissue samples to identify, on a cellular level, what is going on. This is often done to consider or confirm the possibility of cancer. Obtaining a biopsy is not such a big problem if the area of concern is a visible target such as a skin lesion

Modified barium swallow

An MBS is an x-ray test that visualizes the structure and function of the mouth, pharynx, and esophagus. Movement of foods and fluids of various textures is observed as they pass through the phases of swallowing. This identifies both structural problems, such as obstruction and narrowing, and the functional problem of aspiration (food or fluids leaking into the lungs). Specific recommendations can be made about swallowing abilities and the safest dietary consistencies.

or visible lump. The area is injected with an anesthetic.

Cases where the target is deep within the body are more complicated. Tissue samples of the breast, liver, and bone to name a few can be obtained with a needle through the skin. Other internal organs can be accessed by endoscopy (described next). These procedures may need sedating medicines and/or numbing medicine on the skin. There will be post-procedure discomfort and possibly a small wound. Again, patient cooperation with positioning and stillness is required.

Endoscopies

Endoscopy is the type of evaluation that uses a scope of some sort to be inserted through a body part to directly visualize the area in question or to obtain a sample for biopsy of lung or stomach. This is done through the mouth to look into the bronchi or the stomach, or up the rectum to see the colon. This is usually done in the hospital under sedation, and the patient sleeps through the test. The after-effects are usually limited to the sedation medication or some post-procedure soreness.

STEP 4: TREATMENT

It's important to note that many problems exist that have no clear diagnosis. At any point along the way, patients may choose to consult with (or be referred to) specialists for either the diagnosis or the treatment plan. Alternatively, the "ruling out" of ominous causes may be a sufficiently satisfactory outcome. In those cases, symptom management may be the next course of action.

Medications

Medications are a mainstay of medical treatment. They are used in vast numbers by people living at home, in the hospital, or in rehab and long-term care settings. They are prescribed to treat medical conditions, come in many forms, are given by many routes, and are ordered in several types of schedules. The issue of med compliance—is this person taking all medication in the manner that it was prescribed?—is always of great concern, but the more medications taken the greater the likelihood of errors or problems.

What follows is a review of the issues surrounding the use of medications in various settings and the special considerations needed for the very old. This review includes the components of medication orders and their issues as they relate to those of advanced age, as well as strategies to improve or maintain med compliance.

Categories of Medications

Short-term medications, such as antibiotics, are meant to treat an acute illness. They are given one or more times a day for a specific length of time, with the goal of eradicating the problem.

Long-term medications are prescribed for chronic conditions such as high blood pressure, heart disease, diabetes, and COPD. These are taken either one or more times a day for an indefinite period of time. These medications may have changes in dosages depending upon individual response or changing status.

PRNs are medications that are taken on an intermittent basis to treat or relieve symptoms. PRN is a Latin phrase—*pro re nata*—that translates to "as needed for," and these medications usually have a frequency interval, such as "every four hours PRN pain." Medications for pain, nausea, and cough fall into this category. PRN medications can be taken occasionally or as often as several times a day. It is a good idea to write down how often these are taken.

Over-the-counter (OTC) refers to medicine that a person can purchase without a prescription. For some reason many people seem to think that these meds are somehow safer than prescriptions. This is definitely not the case. In fact, many medications formerly requiring prescriptions are now available OTC. These self-serve medications often complicate care for many reasons. Sometimes elders usse them for the wrong thing, in the wrong way, causing more problems, such as using ibuprofen for the pain that is from an ulcer, not arthritis, or mixing it with alcohol and blood thinners. These meds miss the safety measure of a pharmacist checking for drug interactions with prescription meds. There is no record of history of use or response, and the elders' memory of when they take these types of medications can be vague or faulty. As a safety precaution, these meds should be included on all home med lists and brought to medical appointments.

MEDICATION ORDERS AND MONITORING

In medication orders, to ensure that the medication is correctly administered, healthcare professionals use "The Five Rights":

1. the Right Person

2. the Right Medication

3. in the Right Dose

4. by the Right Route

5. at the Right Time.

In a hospital or other institutionalized setting, the identification wristband is the protection for *the Right Person* part, so it's essential to make sure the ancient one is wearing the wristband all the time.

In terms of selecting the *Right Medication*, the very name of a medication can be confusing. Sometimes meds are referred to by their brand name; other times the generic name is used. Healthcare providers and institutions may be inconsistent. If there are questions, ask the doctor, nurse, or pharmacist. Try to make sure that the medicine names listed with instructions for home medication match the names on the actual bottles.

The *Right Dose* can also be a challenge. Sometimes dosages vary from the general directions to the ones on the medication bottles. You may need to give 30 milligrams of a liquid but the pharmacist has given you only a 10 milligram measuring spoon, so you'll need to use it three times. (Note that ancient ones may be used to teaspoons instead of metric measurements, which can complicate things even further.) Be sure to double-check all numbers before administering any doses.

When I work with patients I encourage them to ask the nurse or at-home caregiver for the name and dose of each med, just to be sure it seems right. A confident and capable nurse or caregiver should never resist or feel distrusted by this interest. Medication errors happen in institutions as well as in people's homes. There is good reason for caution.

The *Right Route* refers to the way the medication gets into the body. Possibilities include

- by mouth, in the form of tablet, capsule, or liquid;

- injected into flesh, muscle, or vein, with a needle or small tube;

- applied topically through the skin (as a cream, lotion, gel, or ointment) or as drops for the eyes or ears;

- inhaled into lungs, by way of pocket inhaler or nebulizer; or

- inserted into the rectum or vagina with a suppository or cream.

Always make sure that route is clear before administering any medication.

The *Right Time* refers to the schedule for the meds. It describes the number of times, and at what time, the med is to be taken and for how long. Examples include once daily, three times a day before meals, every twelve hours, at bedtime, for ten days, and so forth. Do not stop administering a medication such as an antibiotic prematurely without discussing it first with the prescriber.

There should be ongoing monitoring for medications of any form. Particular awareness is needed of changes in the use of PRNs, as it may reflect a change in the underlying problem. For instance, when an elder starts going through a bottle of pain meds at a rapid rate, further evaluation may be needed, along with a different approach for treatment, such as the addition of physical therapy.

If there is a pattern to taking the as-needed meds, it may be wise to add them to the scheduled meds. For example if a pain med is taken in the morning and afternoon as needed, put these in the appropriate spot in a pillbox (see strategy list below). This will not only improve comfort, it can also improve safety by minimizing interaction with a whole bottle of pills.

STRATEGIES TO IMPROVE OR MAINTAIN MED COMPLIANCE

The improper use of many medications can—and often does—have dire consequences. Families or caregivers of ancient ones can take steps such as the following to help keep things on the right track.

- Keep a list of all medications and bring it to all medical appointments. It should include all medications, prescriptions, vitamins and supplements and over-the-counter drugs. Just as the medical record is updated (hopefully) with each change, make sure the elder's own list is kept current. Many people take a list of medications to their office appointment only to have the dosages and frequency of the medications changed. The list can get very confusing with multiple cross–outs, so start with a fresh list as often as necessary. Make sure it is legible, and put a date on the list so you can tell that it's the most recent version.

- Have all prescriptions filled at the same pharmacy. This step serves as an extra check to verify that all the medications the elderly person is taking are compatible. Chances for unwanted interactions increase with each added medicine. Store pharmacists are excellent resources for reviewing concerns about any of the medications (both prescription and OTC), including potential drug interactions.

- For patients with hearing, visual, or cognitive impairments, make an effort to ensure that the patients understand the changes. Ask providers to write down and date all directions in big letters.

- Keep up with refill schedules. People with multiple medical problems often take up to twenty medications daily. Make sure that all proper medications and associated supplies (e.g., insulin syringes and lancets) are in stock at home. Medications that have been stopped should be put in a different place than active ones.

- Purchase and set up refillable pillboxes with separate compartments for days of the week and times of day. Even people with no memory problems and those who take only a few pills daily should not feel insulted by the suggestion of a pillbox. It is very easy for anyone to forget a dose or to think a dose was forgotten and take an extra one. It is better to play it safe, take the guesswork out of it, and get (and use!) a pillbox. Keep in mind that these do not help with the administration of PRN meds.

- Request a "blister" or "bubble" pack if the pharmacy offers this service. These are cards that contain rows of plastic "bubbles" that each contain a pill. Made up individually by a pharmacist for a patient according to the medical order, the formatting of the cards depends upon the individual medication plan. A row of pills can represent the morning meds and the next row can be the afternoon pills. Or every different card can be a month's supply of one medication, and one pill is removed from the card at a time. No matter how this is structured, it has advantages of ease both in administration and monitoring of compliance. Note that it does not help if the med plan has frequent changes, and there may be an extra charge for the packaging.

- Use technical methods to improve medication compliance. Some machines or automated devices give programmed verbal directions about meds. For instance, at a preset time (e.g., 9:00 A.M.), a recorded voice will say, "It is time for your medication; you need to take your three pills." Similarly, medication dispensers provide recorded reminders and then dispense the meds that have been previously set up. Note that this type of system can be expensive and won't be a good match for everyone.

Even when all of these steps are taken, it's important to review them on a regular basis to make sure the systems are still working. For instance, the successful use of pillboxes still relies on the ancient ones' continued ability to know the time of day as well as the day of week. Elders who develop memory problems may begin to forget the time or date and will need someone to call them to remind them to open the pillbox. At some point in the spectrum of cognitive decline, there will be a point when the elder should have no role in medication beyond accepting the drug, and no reminder or pillbox can change that.

Friends, family, prescribers, and other healthcare workers also need to be aware of potential discrepancies between what medicines have been ordered and what is actually being taken. When medication changes occur based on inaccurate information, the risk of problems increases dramatically, and sorting it all out can require a lot of sleuthing.

Finally, it's important to review the efficacy and ongoing need of the medications with the physicians or other providers who prescribed them. As times goes on, there are many instances when medicines for issues such as high cholesterol, risk for bone fractures, and the progression of dementia have outlived their usefulness. Particularly at the end of life, a reasonable therapeutic approach to discomfort is what could be called the "subtraction plan" of medicine. Careful assessment of the risks and benefits is important in these cases. A thoughtful medication reduction plan can have interesting results. Sometimes on fewer medications, the ancient ones just feel better and their appetite improves. Understanding that an individual's decline is inevitable, medical care shouldn't create problems that are more unpleasant than the disease itself.

Diabetes Medication and Treatment

Diabetes is a common and complicated metabolic disorder that causes unhealthy elevation in blood sugar. This in turn causes damage to blood vessels and organs, predisposing the ancient one to heart, kidney, circulatory, and vision problems. The treatment involves dietary control and often medicines.

There are many kinds of medications to treat diabetes, including pills, as well as varieties of injected insulin that differ in timing of onset, peak effect, and duration. Some patients require two or more injections daily. There may also be a "sliding scale" plan for a scheduled daily dose plus extra insulin when the blood sugars run high as tested with a fingerstick. This is a complicated program that is far too difficult for many ancient ones to be expected to manage. The administration of injections is routine for nurses, but it can be a challenging process for an older person to learn.

Ancient ones who need to give injections must be able to see the lines on the syringe, hold the syringe and medication vial, draw up the proper amount of medicine into the syringe, and understand when to do this. These tasks require a certain amount of cognition, visual acuity, finger dexterity, motivation, and compliance. Also needed is the intestinal fortitude to inject the needle into the patient, even when it's yourself.

Attempts to control high sugars often result in an overshooting of the goal, which causes dangerous low sugars that create malaise, confusion, and blurred vision—not what an elderly, frail person needs. For this reason, the target range of blood sugar for ancient ones often becomes more liberal, especially since the reduction of risk of long-term complications is no longer the primary goal. Cognitive impairment and diabetes is a perilous combination without proper supervision. Be sure to make arrangements as needed so ancient ones don't need to manage this condition on their own.

Life-Sustaining Treatments

The treatment of medical conditions continues with the minimization of symptoms and steps to optimize general function and well-being. However, in some cases the end of life comes quickly or evolves from the events at hand. The following discussion describes the various possible options in life-sustaining treatments. These are the specific treatments for any of the various system failures that may result in death.

CARDIO-PULMONARY RESUSCITATION (CPR)

Cardio-pulmonary resuscitation (CPR) is an emergency intervention that is undertaken when there is no pulse or respirations. If elders remain untreated in this condition, nature will take its course and they will likely be dead in a matter of minutes.

Ideally, CPR is begun at the earliest moment of death: the absence of heartbeat and/or spontaneous breathing. Its goal is revival—bringing the patient back to life—and it is the most extreme example of life-sustaining treatment. The procedure involves compressing the heart forcefully between the breastbone and the spine. If there is a return of spontaneous heartbeat but the person is not breathing, it may be necessary to use mechanical intubation with a ventilator or breathing machine.

CPR is considered to be the standard of care to initiate on all persons regardless of age or status (decapitation is exempt) unless there is a direct and clear order to not do so. The official designation of *DNR* or *Do Not Resuscitate* is for those who choose to avoid this measure. However, the chances of meaningful recovery in a frail elder undergoing CPR are very small, while the chances of pain and injury are almost guaranteed.

MECHANICAL VENTILATION

This is another life-support intervention that is done in the case of respiratory failure, which can occur very suddenly or over several hours. This type of care is often initiated in the emergency room and continued in the intensive care unit (ICU) in a hospital. It can be part of the CPR experience or as a response to severe lung disease.

The patient is intubated, which means that a tube is inserted into the airway through the mouth and then attached to a mechanical ventilator. This is a complex and specialized machine that moves air in and out of the lungs. It limits the patient's ability to eat, talk, and move around.

Whether this is a temporary or permanent situation may not be certain at the onset. Some people will agree to a brief trial of intubation with the expectation they will recover sufficiently to breathe on their own (such as after treatment of pneumonia or during an operation). The timeline of this serious situation is individualized. If improvement does not occur and normal breathing does not resume, there will need to be a discussion of options. Long-term mechanical ventilation may be considered, but it requires specialized settings with ongoing skilled and technical support. If this is not a desired option, the decision can be made to come off the machine and allow death to occur with comfort measures in place. These situations are so much clearer when there are formal advance directives in place that guide the care.

DIALYSIS

Dialysis provides a form of life support for people with kidney failure. This is a high-tech, intermittent but often lifelong treatment that involves filtering the blood of waste products the body can no longer process. Dialysis (or *hemodialysis*) usually requires the patient to go to a specialized unit, three times a week, and plug into a machine, usually through a specially made area under the skin of the forearm. Each treatment lasts approximately four hours. The patient can live life as usual during his or her non-dialysis days. With this in mind, it's important to note that transportation issues are common, and the duration of the ride contributes to the exhaustion level that is common in the elders who undergo this treatment.

Kidney function can decline quickly with an acute illness, but more commonly the changes can take place over years. The discussion about the desire and/or need for dialysis treatment can occur over months, even years, and should certainly be a consideration for advanced directives.

FEEDING TUBES

Feeding tubes are a low-tech, life-support intervention used to maintain nutrition and hydration in a person unable to do so. A feeding tube is used for a variety of reasons. These include

- a sudden inability to swallow due to a new stroke or accident (duration that tube will be needed is unknown at onset);

- an acute illness that has limited the elder's alertness or strength to eat (duration that tube will be needed is expected to be temporary);

- an inability to swallow due to treatment of head and neck cancer (duration that tube will be needed is often temporary);

- an ineffective swallow leading to respiratory infections (based on the progression of the chronic problem overall, worsening can usually be expected and tube-feeding is not temporary); and

- weight loss and weakness from dementia, depression, failure to thrive, or progressive chronic disease (based on the progression of the chronic problem overall, worsening can usually be expected and tube-feeding is not temporary).

Sometimes elders have totally lost the ability to swallow; other times the patient is just bad at it, and eating and drinking are associated with coughing, choking, and other uncomfortable symptoms. Sometimes, an ancient one eats some, but just not enough, and tube feedings are used to supplement the daily intake or just provide fluids.

Even if the overall situation is an emergency, there is time for careful consideration about the question of inserting a feeding tube. It is a simple procedure and the care and maintenance are not difficult, but an elderly person is unlikely to be able to maintain it independently. A pencil-thin flexible tube, fastened to the skin of the abdomen, passes into the stomach. A liquid formula is used to meet the elder's nutritional and fluid needs. The feeding can be done at a slow rate over the whole day, more quickly over fewer hours, or in larger amounts over a half hour several times a day. Medications can also be given this way, either in crushed or liquid form. Water is provided several times throughout the day to meet fluid needs. Both nutrition and fluid intake can be closely monitored and changed in response to activity and physical conditions.

Discussion should include the identification of which problems will improve with better nutrition and which will not. For example, dementia, respiratory disease, and cancer will keep their own course and unpleasant symptoms will persist despite the feeding tube. As this treatment requires cooperation on the part of the patient, it is very difficult to manage this in a confused, anxious, or restless person.

This decision needs to be put in the light of the overall goals of care. Considering the elder's current status and expected prognosis, think carefully about whether this may be a time when comfort measures, such as focusing on pleasurable activities, should surpass concerns about nutrition. If the patient is incapacitated, and there is no advanced directive in place about the use of feeding tubes, then family members or the health care agent must work with healthcare professions to consider this option.

This kind of life support can be a good long-term solution for ancient ones who are otherwise healthy but simply unable to swallow, enabling them to live several more years of life. Alternatively it can maintain the life in a frail and profoundly impaired elder until there is eventual multisystem failure, which may not be the type of plan that anyone wants.

Intravenous Hydration

Intravenous hydration tools (IVs) are commonly used for administering medications when the oral route is not indicated because of the elder's condition or the specific type of med. However, when an ancient one cannot or will not take oral fluids, then IVs for hydration become a life-sustaining intervention. This is very helpful in the short term during times of acute illness, particularly when there is too much lethargy or symptoms are too severe for the elder to maintain sufficient fluid status. It is not a long-term solution to chronic poor intake.

A simple IV in the arm treats dehydration by providing fluids with small amounts of salt and sugar, but nothing in terms of nutrition. With an IV in place, the total lack of nutrition is tolerable for at least a few days while waiting for improvements in overall condition (when drinking can be resumed), or while coming up with a more long-term plan, such as comfort measures or the placement of a feeding tube.

For an elderly person, IV therapy, as simple as it is, takes its toll. The placement of the tube into the arm must be changed every three to five days, to minimize the risk of inflammation and infection. Ancient veins are delicate and skin is thin, dislodging of the tube is common, and bruises are numerous. Consequently, the benefits should always be weighed against the disadvantages.

* * *

All of these life-sustaining treatments have their usefulness in the population at large, and some very old persons want no limitations on these treatments in the event of severe or sudden illness. The important thing is to make sure elders and their agents understand the issues and know (and record) the ancient one's preferences. Remember that when there are no advance directives to guide medical care, the standard is to proceed with all of the above described interventions as they are deemed to be needed.

Chapter Seven

Basic Physical Issues

There are hundreds—if not thousands—of medical diagnoses and countless combinations of problems. Trying to sort out health problems diagnosis by diagnosis is extremely difficult and confusing. I find that reducing medical problems to a few basic issues makes the situation more manageable for elders, caregivers, and families. In this chapter I have chosen six basic issues, crossing diagnostic lines, that have important implications for the well-being of elderly folks:

- neuroworks (alertness, orientation, and attitude);

- dysphagia (difficulty swallowing);

- cardiac and respiratory issues;

- fluid balance;

- elimination (urinary and bowel issues); and

- pain.

This chapter also includes a few stories to illustrate the interplay of physiological issues.

Neuroworks: Alertness, Orientation, and Attitude

The nervous system is a magnificently complex and wonderful design. The brain is mapped out so that there are specific locations that are clearly responsible for particular functions. Consequently, there are predictable deficits resulting from damage to corresponding areas. The components of neurologic function that relate to mental status are described more fully in upcoming chapters.

Disorders of the neurological system are sadly common and manifest on a continuum, from function to dysfunction, depending on the extent of damage and the body's ability to respond to or overcome the injury. While healthcare providers understand much of the brain and its activity, there still remain great mysteries.

Neurological problems can be sudden and severe or have a gradual onset and subtle symptoms. Regardless of cause, issues involving function, comfort, and quality of life are very similar, and the ancient one will need a plan to help address the individual goals.

The sudden neurological problems are mainly vascular and result from abnormal bleeding or clotting. One example is *cerebral vascular accident* (CVA or commonly called a *stroke*), which creates functional deficits related to the area injured. This interruption of blood flow can occur from a cerebral hemorrhage (a brain bleed); from a blood clot (thrombus) that develops within the brain slowly, bit by bit; or from an embolus that floats in from elsewhere in the body, often the heart.

Some strokes are the classic type, with a one-sided weakness, called *hemiparesis,* and facial droop, but there are many varieties. Some strokes are fatal immediately, while others result in dysfunction that is incompatible with life because it causes the elders to lose their ability to either breathe and/or swallow nourishment. In those cases, there will be decisions about comfort measures and life support.

Ancient ones who suffer from nonlethal strokes, on the other hand, benefit from as much rehabilitation as feasible. Duration of symptoms and return of function depend upon the location and severity of the injury. Functional improvements are hard to predict; ancient ones who have suffered a stroke may have complete recovery or persistent dysfunction.

Transient ischemic attacks (*TIA*) cause stroke-like symptoms (e.g., weakness; loss of function of body parts; or trouble speaking, comprehending, or seeing) that develop and then resolve completely within a twenty-four-hour period. These can be considered a warning sign that there is risk for more stroke activity. Such alarms give the patient and primary care physician a chance to do whatever is possible to minimize risks for further stroke. This can include blood pressure control, cholesterol and diabetic control, or anticoagulation if indicated. This is also a time to include advance directives as part of the discussion.

There are many neurological diseases that cause a variety of incapacitating symptoms, such as Alzheimer's disease, Parkinson's disease, and multiple sclerosis. Cancer is a group of diseases that can either start or spread to the brain, causing pain and functional impairment. Brain injuries occurring from trauma can cause a wide range of symptoms.

Many neurological conditions result in physical weakness, communication impairment, and/or cognitive decline. Often there are progressive qualities that cause an ongoing degeneration and dysfunction. Severe problems can result in major debility or death.

Before we move on, let's take a look at a few stories to illustrate the idea that similar issues and challenges exist in people with different diagnoses. This reinforces the concept that

Aphasia

Aphasia is a brain disorder that affects communication. This occurs when the language center of the brain is damaged by a CVA (cerebral vascular accident, or stroke), an illness, an injury, or a tumor.

- *Expressive aphasia* is more common and impairs the ability to express thoughts. With expressive aphasia, verbal communication can be very difficult, and there is much individual variability in the extent of the disorder. Sometimes it may be as minor as word-finding trouble or as severe as total lack of meaningful speech. This is not a problem with the muscles of the mouth or the breath needed to form sound, although those can coexist with aphasia; it is an issue that stems from the brain itself.

- *Receptive aphasia* makes it difficult for patients to understand verbal or written communication that is directed at them. It is not a hearing or vision problem; it is a language comprehension problem.

Both forms of this disorder are extremely frustrating. Ancient ones may suddenly feel as though they are living where they don't speak the language. Communication can turn into charades or guessing games. Patience and diligence are needed to work out effective communication strategies. Speech therapists can help patients address these issues and work toward improved communication.

healthcare needs to be aimed at these functional issues with as much attention as providers give to the treatment of individual lists of diagnoses and diseases. It is the interplay and balance of these complex issues that supports quality of life

In the following story, brothers Jim and Tom have differing neurological disorders but both struggle with similar issues of weakness and swallowing troubles, which lead to fluid balance problems.

Jim and Tom

Jim had Parkinson's disease, a chronic and progressive neurologic disorder. It didn't cause too much trouble at first. He experienced some stiffness, but with medication he led a normal life and a happy retirement. In his mid-eighties, however, things just seemed to speed up, and he was having greater difficulty getting around. He needed help getting dressed, and he was prone to falls. He began to require more medication to keep symptoms at bay. Scared by his slowing reflexes, he sold his car.

Jim began to drool, and he developed a cough. It took him a very long time to eat, and he often choked when he did. He developed swallowing troubles, which led to recurrent respiratory infections. Each episode left him weaker.

Jim worked with a speech therapist to prevent these infections. He was advised to change his diet, including softer foods and thickened liquids. This caused problems because he didn't like the thick liquids, so he cut down on fluids. If he was very thirsty he cheated and drank plain water instead of a thicker liquid, but as a result he coughed and coughed. He began to develop chronic dehydration and became progressively weaker. He then developed low blood pressure that went even lower when he stood up (*orthostatic hypotension*). It is not surprising that he had a few falls. Most of the time he had just a few bumps and bruises, but one time he injured his arm with a deep laceration and needed stitches.

As Jim received the stitches, the medical team realized that he was dehydrated. He was admitted to the hospital and given IV fluids. However, the fluids were too much for his system, and he developed fluid overload, which resulted in excess fluid accumulating in his lower legs and lungs. He ended up needing diuretics to drain the fluid away, in spite of the fact that he was admitted with dehydration.

Jim's brother, Tom, was just a little younger but was in much better shape. He could golf, drive, and chase around his grandkids. His diabetes and high blood pressure didn't bother him. Then, however, he had a big stroke (CVA). Although the nature of the neurologic problem was very different from Jim's Parkinson's disease, the challenges were similar. They both needed help with activities of daily living (ADLs). In addition to left-sided weakness, Tom had trouble swallowing. This led to both dehydration (because he too hated the thickened liquids) and aspiration pneumonia (because he just did what he wanted and continued to drink thin liquids). These actions also contributed to progressive weakness and subsequent falls. Recovering from his stroke was a big challenge, and instead of optimizing his recovery, his choice to discount advice resulted in an overall declining condition.

The story of these brothers shows how one thing leads to another as the primary problem of neurological dysfunction evolved into difficulty with basic survival by compromising eating and drinking, resulting in breathing problems and dehydration. As these stories illustrate, the complexity of problems and the interconnectedness of symptoms and treatments leave individuals and their families a bit mystified about how to manage. At this point, it really is about managing the issues, because the root of the problem is not going to go away.

Dysphagia and Aspiration: Down the Wrong Pipe

Most people take for granted the way food, fluid, and medications get into their bodies. We take food and fluid into our mouth and down it goes. Yet consider the sequential activities that must occur once we get the food to the mouth, chew it into small pieces, and then swallow it so it goes down the throat. After the food or fluids get into the esophagus, having successfully bypassed the airway, things become automatic and down it goes toward the stomach. It is here that the material—food, fluids, and meds—are able to be of use. Nutrients, water, and medicine will start being absorbed, a process that continues throughout the gastrointestinal (GI) tract.

Aging causes troubles in every part of this process. *Dysphagia*, which means difficulty swallowing, is a common problem in the elderly. They can have trouble chewing food, forming the chewed food into a cohesive blob, and getting the blob from the front of the mouth to the back of the throat. This part of the process is a voluntary activity. Ancient ones need to have a level of awareness and coordination to manage swallowing while at the same time breathing or, harder still, talking. Problems in this area are very common in those with cognitive loss. The progressive disorientation of dementia causes a set-up for swallowing problems. People are easily distracted and disorganized in the initial motor planning, and they have poor swallowing abilities.

Aspiration results when liquids or solids end up in the airway and in the lungs. In the severe and obvious form, aspiration involves choking, with the classic, dramatic picture of a

Dysphagia Diet

Dietary modification in terms of textures is often advised to prevent aspiration. The foods may need to be chopped and moistened, ground, or even pureed. Fluids, on the other hand, need to be thickened to make them easier to manage. This is done by using a special starch powder to achieve the desired consistency. This can be added to a beverage of choice or can be bought as a pre-thickened liquid. The fluid consistency recommendation can range from a nectar-thick beverage to honey-thick or syrup consistency, or for severe dysphagia, a pudding thickness that barely seems liquid.

Unfortunately, these restrictions may be unappealing, and if the ancient ones refuse them, or reduce overall intake, insufficient fluids may lead to a predisposition toward dehydration. Making matters worse, these thickened liquids are not effective at quenching thirst, so they can leave patients unsatisfied, often pleading for water. This can be a big dilemma for families who need to decide whether to minimize risk of aspiration versus pleasure and/or risk of dehydration. Many people choose the greater risk of aspiration in order to improve the chances to get the ancient one to eat or drink something appealing and satisfying.

speechless, throat-clutching, panicked person struggling for life. In this case, the Heimlich maneuver, an emergency choking remedy, can release the chunk of food caught in the person's airway.

More common is the subtle form of aspiration, which ranges from coughing or throat clearing during and after meals to "wet voice" quality to eyes watering at mealtime. Called *silent aspiration*, this can go on at a low level for months without detection. Weight loss is a common result, as eating becomes a less than pleasant event. Chronic cough can also occur, with frequent respiratory infections that may be hard to resolve.

Speech therapists can conduct a swallowing evaluation and, based upon these findings, make recommendations about the safest textures of foods patients should eat. Therapy may include strategies to maximize function, such as positioning properly during eating and drinking, changing food textures, and eating at most alert times.

Even with all these measures in place, many individuals are at ongoing risk of aspiration. The concern for weight loss, malnutrition, weakness, and recurrent respiratory infections can prompt consideration of tube feeding or the clarified plan of supportive care and comfort measures, with the expectation of ongoing decline.

Cardiac and Respiratory Issues: Beats and Breath

HEART TROUBLE

The heart is responsible for the pumping of the blood, which carries oxygen to all parts of the body. The healthy heart is a highly synchronized organ that contracts and relaxes in rhythmic regularity without fail. Advancing age causes assorted problems in the heart. Insufficient blood to the heart itself due to narrowing of coronary arteries causes chest pain or heart attacks. Problems with the valves within the heart can cause dizziness, shortness of breath, or chest pain.

Arrhythmias or irregular heart rhythm can be asymptomatic or can have severe complications. *Atrial fibrillation* (*A Fib*), is a common arrhythmia in the elderly that affects the heart's rhythm. *A Fib* refers to an irregular pattern of uncoordinated beating and ineffective pumping. The rate can be rapid, producing dizziness, fatigue, and heart failure. Treatment is required because incomplete emptying of the heart's chambers may cause pooling of the blood with a subsequent formation of clots, and a clot that moves through the heart into the brain will result in a common type of stroke or cerebral vascular accident (CVA). The treatment of atrial fibrillation is aimed at normalizing the rate and rhythm of the heart, and preventing blood clots with anticoagulation.

Congestive heart failure (CHF) is a common malady in the very old. This condition of the weakening of the heart muscle involves both acute and chronic components. Shortness of breath and cough are common symptoms and can worsen suddenly. Subtle weight gain, as well as swelling of the feet, ankles, and legs, can be early warning signs of fluid build-up. Close observation and frequent monitoring, including daily weight checks, can prevent flare-ups, a common cause of hospitalizations. There are numerous medications that help control symptoms, but these need frequent adjustments to prevent complications.

Many of these conditions coexist in older persons, which makes it difficult to sort out which problem is causing the symptom. This is why shortness of breath is a symptom that merits careful evaluation.

Oxygen

Supplemental oxygen can be used to fortify the air, which is only 20 percent oxygen, to help raise the amount of oxygen in the elder's blood. This extra oxygen is needed to treat some kinds of heart and lung disease.

Supplemental oxygen is a gas that is administered from a tank or a machine called a *concentrator* and is carried through tubing or face mask that has a two-pronged tube called a *cannula*, which goes slightly into each nostril. This type of extra oxygen is dosed as if it were a medication. The directions are given in terms of liter flow, often with a range, such as 2 to 4 liters a minute. Oxygen can be provided continuously or on an intermittent basis for episodic shortness of breath.

In individuals with healthy lungs, the force that drives breath is excess carbon dioxide. Humans are prompted to breathe because of the need to get rid of excess carbon dioxide by exhaling. People with lung disorders, however, grow accustomed to higher levels of carbon dioxide in their blood. Their impulse to breathe comes from the need to inhale. When there is too much oxygen in the system from high-flow supplemental oxygen, the stimulus for breathing is taken away and patients lose the drive to breathe. There can be problems with the dosing, and it is possible to overdose on oxygen, with dire consequences. Ancient ones who overdose on oxygen may get sleepy, confused, or agitated; they can pass out and, potentially, die. Remember that when it comes to oxygen therapy, some is good but more is not better.

RESPIRATORY DYSFUNCTION

Breathe in, breathe out—respiration goes on and on, minute after minute, day after day, starting at birth and continuing for as long as we live. Everything we do depends upon that breath, every movement and every thought. The respiratory system is responsible for taking the air into the lungs, where the vital exchange of gases takes place. Oxygen is inhaled and carbon dioxide is exhaled. Every cell in the body needs oxygen and a sufficient delivery (circulatory) system to function properly.

Breathing problems are very common in the elderly. Often these problems involve the narrowing of the air passages, which makes the inflow and the outflow difficult. This causes an increased effort to breathe, which in turn causes the person to wheeze. When aging lungs lose their ability to process air, it causes shortness of breath.

Chronic obstructive pulmonary disease (COPD) is a common and progressive form of respiratory dysfunction. It includes *chronic bronchitis*, with frequent productive cough, and *emphysema,* a condition that results in decreased gas exchange within the lungs. Advanced age and cigarette smoking are the main causes of emphysema, which involves a chronic, often progressive, shortness of breath.

Individuals with chronic lung disease are prone to respiratory infections because of impaired defenses, and when they have an infection, their overall respiratory status declines. Early symptoms include difficulties breathing with exertion, such as climbing stairs or strenuous activity. As lung function worsens, there is more shortness of breath with less exertion, and a longer time is needed to recover to normal breathing. Severe disease causes markedly decreased activity tolerance, and breathlessness can limit talking and eating.

Treatments involve inhaled medicines both on a regular and as-needed basis while steroids are used for flare-ups. Severe COPD exacerbations are a common cause of hospitalizations. It is not surprising that these breathing problems and anxiety are close companions, as one increases the other.

Pneumonia is an infection in the lungs, and before antibiotics became widely available, it was a frequent cause of death. Today, while there are many treatments and most patients fully recover, pneumonia is still a serious illness. It can be the main problem or occur as a complication of other medical or surgical hospitalizations. It can also be due to generalized debility with or without swallowing problems. Pneumonia is often seen in end-of-life situations as the last chapter of chronic disease.

Sylvia's story, which appears next, highlights the issues that result from the combined effects of heart and lung problems. These are serious problems with inherent risks from treatment, and much of the medical treatment is aimed at minimizing these complications of care.

Sylvia

It was no wonder that she had a cough. Sylvia had smoked for sixty-five years and coughed for at least the last twenty. Shortness of breath limited her activities, and it was getting worse. First she had trouble on the stairs, later walking, and now she found that telling a long story was a breathless chore. Her activities were being slowly controlled and restricted by her worsening symptoms.

Sylvia had both chronic lung and heart disease, COPD, coronary artery disease, atrial fibrillation, and congestive heart failure. Her symptoms were the result of difficulties getting the air into the lungs and getting the oxygen from the air into the blood. Her heart had trouble pumping the blood to all the places in her body it needed to go. Occasionally, fluid would move out of the blood and into the tissues, where it accumulated in her legs and lungs, leaving her weaker and more short of breath.

Sylvia took a variety of medications, including some to strengthen and slow the heart, lower blood pressure, open airways, decrease inflammation, remove extra fluid, replace potassium, and thin the blood. Several times a day, there were pills, liquids, and inhalers, and when her sugars went up she took insulin injections too. She was on continuous oxygen and needed a special diet. Her weight needed to be monitored daily. When her struggle to breathe was too much, her stress escalated, so she would take anti-anxiety meds.

Sylvia sometimes might eat too much salt or forget or mismanage her meds. Her weight would creep up and she would develop shortness of breath, coughing, and swelling in feet and ankles. She had too much fluid in her tissues and not enough in her blood vessels. Her doctor would prescribe more diuretics, which made her pee day and night. The frequent trips to the toilet were tiresome and the sleep disruption was exhausting.

At this point Sylvia was as much at risk from progressive weakness as she was from her medical issues. Her various meds caused a drop in blood pressure and occasional dizziness. Sometimes she would restrict fluids to get a break from bathroom trips. This may have seemed sensible, but it actually worsened her condition by adding mild dehydration to an already strained body. Her weakened state and nocturnal perambulations put her at great risk for falls.

Her hospitalizations due to shortness of breath were often complicated stays. While she was being treated for the various components of her illness, including heart failure and fluid overload, lung disease, and pneumonia, she also suffered from the complications often encountered from these ailments and their medications, such as bleeding and clotting problems, diarrhea, and mental status changes. After Sylvia was medically stabilized in the hospital, she would then need a rehab stay to regain the strength lost during illness and sort out any of the residual issues (medical, functional, or social) before returning home.

FLUID BALANCE: HIGH TIDE AND DRY

Fluid balance is precarious with very old people. Understanding the dynamics of fluids in the body can help in the early identification of symptoms and in maintaining functional status.

Fluids are located in three general places in the body:

- in the blood vessels, maintaining blood pressure and circulation;

- in the tissues, surrounding and nourishing the cells; and, mostly

- in the cells, allowing proper functioning of organs.

The balance of fluids within these spaces is very important for physiologic functioning and good health.

The initial medical evaluation of a person with suspected fluid imbalance is straightforward. A healthcare provider can easily identify problems by means of simple blood and urine tests. Even when the cause of the problem is not so obvious, providers can treat dehydration or fluid overload even before they identify the cause.

Dehydration

Fluid normally goes into the body through the mouth by way of food and liquid intake. Fluid comes out many more ways: in urine, stool, sweat, wound drainage, bleeding, nasal discharge, vomitus and sputum, and through breathing as vapor. In fact, a surprising amount of fluid (at least a liter a day) is lost through normal breathing. Many illnesses produce symptoms (increased respiratory rate, loose stools, vomiting, or fever) that result in fluid loss, and the balance will be tipped, resulting in dehydration.

Dehydration occurs because too little fluid goes in and/or too much comes out. Like so many other problems, dehydration can be abrupt and dramatic, as with a bout of a stomach virus, or it can occur slowly due to insufficient intake and reach a critical mass without a clear precipitating event. There is a "chicken and egg" quality to these issues, as it can be hard to tell if the problem is dehydration or if the problem is caused by dehydration.

Often elderly people aren't aware of the decrease in thirst, which only contributes to the problem. Many ancient ones are also bothered by urinary frequency, either due to the natural aging process or because of diuretics or fluid pills that keep folks running to the bathroom. As a result, they may consciously decide to decrease fluid intake to minimize trips to the bathroom.

Dehydration can create a cascade of problems. Blood volume and blood pressure is maintained by the presence of an adequate fluid status. The lack of fluids that occurs in even mild dehydration will decrease volume within the blood vessels and may result in low or unstable blood pressure, especially with positional changes. *Orthostatic hypotension* is the formal term for the drop in blood pressure that occurs when the person moves from the lying position to the sitting or standing position. This movement can produce a woozy, lightheaded feeling, and a fall can occur.

The kidneys are always working to maintain the optimum concentrations of fluids and salts, such as sodium and potassium. These concentrations change in the state of dehydration, and toxins can build up in the bloodstream. This can cause lethargy and confusion, prompting errors in judgment and falls.

Dehydration will also impair the body's ability to metabolize certain medications, potentially causing a dangerous build up of these chemicals. This can further impair kidney function, and so the downward cycle continues. Urine becomes more concentrated and thereby more caustic, predisposing ancient ones to urinary tract discomfort, infection, and even mental status changes. Constipation is caused in part or worsened by insufficient fluid intake; stools are retained and more moisture is absorbed out of the stools, causing them to be hard and dry.

Excess Fluid

The balance can also tip in the other direction, and the body can retain fluids in amounts that are in excess to its needs. Fluids build up for many reasons, such as heart, vascular, or kidney disease; metabolic conditions, such as low thyroid; nutritional deficiencies; or medication side effects. Sodium restriction is important to keep swelling at bay.

Fluid retention is often a recurrent or chronic situation that needs monitoring and management. This fluid, which is in the tissues outside the vessels and around the cells, will usually show up in different ways. Most commonly, there will be swelling or edema of the feet, ankles, or legs, or in the backside if the ancient one is bedridden.

The first response to this swelling of the feet should be to elevate them. Feet up on a foot-

Intake and Output (I&O)

Intake and output is a way to monitor an ancient one's general fluid status. During worrisome times of sickness, what goes in the body and what comes out can be measured to see if fluids are retained or if the body is heading toward dehydration. This is done routinely in hospital and rehab settings, but it can be done at home as well. The intake part is easier to keep track of, with running volumes of beverages and watery food, such as soup. An effective amount of daily fluid intake is usually about 2.5 liters a day.

The output part is more complicated. Urine can be measured in a urinal for men; either gender can use a "hat," a plastic toilet insert that allows for urine measurement. For incontinent elders, measurements of output are estimated in terms of small, medium, and large. The attentive caregiver will be able to notice these differences, as well as color and odor changes of urine.

Alternatively, scant or dark urine output, a very strong odor, or a dry pad can alert caregivers to dehydration. The I&O never balances perfectly because there are many immeasurable fluid losses in the vapor exhaled, in sweat, and in stools, but this information helps identify trends in the fluid status. The output should be within a liter of the input.

stool or hassock are good, but elevation above the level of the heart is even better. This can be done in a recliner, or in bed or on a couch with the feet up on pillows. It can also help to compress the legs using light support stockings or tight-squeezing wraps. For optimum benefit, the patient should put these on before arising from bed, when legs are the most slender. The tighter the compression, the more difficult they are to apply, and elders often need assistance. Part of routine care is to check swollen legs for the development of breaks in the skin or signs of infection, such as increased redness or warmth.

Shortness of breath and cough are symptoms of fluid overload when there is an accumulation of fluid in the lungs. People with severe shortness of breath are frequently hospitalized for this due to congestive heart failure. Diuretics (fluid-reducing pills) are used to help rid the body of excess fluid, and they may be prescribed in both emergency and everyday situations.

Patients who are still living in their own home or with family members can monitor their own fluid status using the common household scale. They can take their weight first thing in the morning after peeing, which will alert them to rapid gaining of weight due to fluid retention. A fluid overload may show as a gain of three pounds in a day or five pounds over two days. An early awareness of this problem can head off impending troubles. Again, this is something patients should report to their primary care physicians. Alternatively this may be done in a hospital or rehab center after an acute episode.

Whenever there is concern for problems with fluid status, healthcare providers can follow a simple method of assessment. The daily measurement of intake and output (I&O) can provide a good deal of information about fluid status.

Elimination
TO PEE OR NOT TO PEE

Doing number one, urinating, peeing, tinkling, voiding, passing water, or *taking a leak* are all terms for the passing of liquid waste products from the body. Again, aging causes problems in this department as well. These problems can be related to pathology, on a continuum of aging, or to medication's side effects. But elders may be reluctant to discuss such matters due to embarrassment, shame, or ignorance of treatment options.

Urinary Frequency
Urinary frequency is extremely common. This is often a result of aging and/or medication. It is often a reason people stay home: to be near the bathroom. When planning an outing, check out the bathroom opportunities in advance, and make plans accordingly. Never miss an opportunity to use the bathroom when on the outing. An incontinent pad may also be advisable, just in case, to provide extra security. Be sure to take a spare to be prepared for accidents.

Incontinence
It can be embarrassing for elders to admit urinary incontinence. This is the partial or complete loss of control of urination. Symptoms range from occasional but predictable leakage (from laughing, coughing, or a long car ride), constant dribbling, or a regular flood. Some people feel that this is an inevitable situation in old age, but that's not necessarily true. A urologist can help evaluate and manage the problem. Even if there isn't a cure for incontinence, possible treatments include medications, physical therapy, high-tech devices, and procedures that can improve symptoms.

Coping with urinary incontinence is a constant struggle. There are no days off or holidays from the diligence needed to maintain skin integrity. As mentioned, thorough cleaning is needed, followed by a barrier cream or ointment. This will leave a layer of protection to keep the urine and stool off the skin. Great improvements have been made in the quality of incontinent products, and there is a vast array of supplies in stores and online to meet any need.

Urinary Tract Infections

A common problem in the elderly is *urinary tract infection* (UTI). This potentially serious illness can cause urinary symptoms of burning, urgency, or frequency; new or worsening incontinence; or a foul odor. There may be constitutional symptoms of malaise, fever, chills, nausea, and vomiting, or mental status changes of confusion or lethargy. These symptoms can come on suddenly or creep up over days. Report any of these symptoms to the primary care provider. This is a common reason elderly persons end up in doctor offices and hospitals and is also a common hospital-acquired infection.

Urinary tract infections are diagnosed by urine sample for urinalysis and culture and are treated with antibiotics. Resolution may be quick and simple, or infections may become chronic or recurrent. Recurrent infections and multiple antibiotic treatments can result in resistant germs and the development of so-called "superbugs." This trend calls for judicious antibiotic usage, with an awareness that urine tests can indicate an infection with absolutely no symptoms. Antibiotics should be avoided in the absence of symptoms; however, careful monitoring for the development of progressive symptoms is indicated.

Urinary Retention

Incomplete bladder emptying or urinary retention can be an insidious problem. It can be a complication of diabetes, a common side effect of mediation, or an enlargement of the prostate gland in men. Pain and recent surgery can predispose elders to this problem. Urinary retention can occur suddenly, with the complete cessation of urination for a period of time. This is likely to prompt unpleasant sensations of bladder distention. More common is the chronically full bladder with overflow urination. In this situation, there may be frequent urination of small amounts without completely emptying the bladder. This is a set-up for infection and can lead to kidney problems if progressive. A catheter will be needed.

A *urinary catheter* is used when urine needs to be collected directly from the bladder. This

Urinary Catheters

An indwelling urinary catheter is a small tube that is inserted into the bladder through the urethra. It is held in place by a small balloon filled with water near the inside tip of the catheter within the bladder. A tube connects the catheter to a collection bag (either a leg bag that fits inside trousers or a bigger, bedside bag). The drainage bag is easily emptied of collected urine through a valve. These catheters are often used temporarily until the need is over. This is commonly called a *Foley Catheter*, named for the inventor.

A *straight cath* describes the insertion of a tube through the urethra into the bladder; the urine is drained and the tube is removed. This is done as a one-shot deal to get a sterile specimen, to check out how much urine is actually in the bladder, or just to empty it because, for some reason, urine is being temporarily retained in the bladder.

These procedures are usually performed by nurses, are done at the bedside, and require sterile technique.

A *suprapubic catheter* is used when there is ongoing need for a catheter. This is a fairly simple surgical procedure, where a tube is inserted through the abdomen into the bladder, and from there it is the same as the indwelling type in terms of tubing and collection. Its main advantage is that the insertion site is away from the "dirtier" parts of the body. This decreases risk of infection by minimizing the opportunities for fecal contamination.

occurs in acute medical situations when fluid status needs to be accurately monitored, during periods of immobility when toileting is too difficult or too painful to be feasible, when there are wounds in the area that would be contaminated by urine, or for urinary retention.

The down side to all kinds of catheters is that they predispose the person to urinary tract infections. The urinary tract is meant to be a sterile environment, but the catheter provides an easy entry for bacteria to get into the body. Proper technique in the insertion and care of the catheter will minimize but not eliminate the risk of contamination. Hand washing is important before any contact with the catheter, tubing, or collection bag. Efforts should be made to remove the catheter as soon as deemed sensible.

There are often several factors that enter the decision-making process in terms of catheter use. Medical stability, mobility, pain, and discomfort are all issues that play into the need for keeping the catheter in. Convenience is not usually a good enough reason to use a catheter.

However, if the goal of care is comfort and people are willing to accept the risk of serious infection, it may be reasonable to use a catheter to simplify the care or increase the comfort of a bedridden person, especially at the end of life.

THE POOP SCOOP

While *Everybody Poops* is an actual book that has been written for children, *Everybody Wants to Poop* and *Everybody Wants to Talk About Poop* would likely be bestsellers among the ancient ones. Nurses and other caregivers often hear—in graphic detail—the trials and tribulations of elders trying to poop. What success and cause for joy with a good movement!

Regularity is the concept of having at least one soft-formed stool a day. There is both truth and wisdom in the old commercial that says that "Regular is what's regular for you." However, if constipation is what's regular, then there is room for improvement of bowel function.

Bathroom habits can be very ritualized at any age, but this is especially true in the elderly. The ancient ones generally don't get out much, and there is often little variation in their daily routines. These people have lived in their bodies for so long, they often have a good idea of what effect certain foods are likely to do to their bowel function.

Constipation

Constipation and fear of it are common problems and motivators for behaviors. As people age, they may

- become less mobile;

- have less thirst;

- drink fewer fluids;

- have a diet with insufficient fiber; and/or

- take multiple prescription medications, which can produce the side effect of constipation.

As a result of these situations, they are often prone to constipation. The best treatment for constipation is prevention approached on multiple levels. As the previous list indicates, fluid intake, food choices, activity, and medications are many of the factors involved in bowel function. Let's take a moment to look at each element in more detail.

• *Fluid intake* includes all beverages and watery food products, such as soup or Jell-O. It is recommended that the average adult consumes eight to ten glasses of fluid on a normal day. In the case of illness, fluids may need to be increased by 25 percent, depending upon symptoms. Illnesses that cause diarrhea or respiratory symptoms, such a labored breathing and cough, can really increase fluid needs.

These fluids should be taken throughout the day. Certain fluids, such as coffee, prune juice, and senna tea, have laxative effects, and these are easy to incorporate into the diet.

• *Diets* should be reasonably high in fiber to help prevent constipation. Fiber or roughage will increase the bulk of the stool. In general, fiber helps alleviate constipation, but in some cases, too much fiber can actually add to the problem by making the stools too large to easily pass. Elders who have lived for many years on a low-fiber diet may not tolerate a sudden change in the amount of fiber in the diet. Symptoms such as abdominal distention, cramps, or bloating can occur. Conversely, if people are used to a lot of fresh fruits and vegetables but no longer have these foods in their diet, their bowels may slow down for want of fiber. Soups, stews, hot grain cereal, and stewed fruit are pleasing and well accepted ways to add good fiber that include high fluid content.

• *Physical activity* is another way to improve bowel function. Exercise in any form is one of the best ways to stay healthy and get bowels moving. Any time activity levels drop off, elders can expect a slowing of bowel function resulting in constipation. To prevent problems during periods of low activity, it may be wise to add a stool softener, modify the diet by adding fiber, and increase fluids. When immobility is the norm, it is very common for elders to require some sort of medication or remedy for improved bowel function.

• *Medications,* both prescription and over the counter, can have side effects of changed bowel function, either constipation or diarrhea. Often these symptoms exist in a person as a tendency, and they are then made worse with the addition of meds. Alert the primary care provider to these tendencies whenever a new medication is being prescribed. There are often other options within the treatment plan that would be helpful in minimizing the risk of side effects. For example, there are numerous medications that treat high blood pressure, but some can worsen constipation, and that merits consideration in choosing a medication. If a specific medication is really needed and there is no better alternative, then the elder must cope with the side effect of constipation. The usual methods of increased fluids, fiber as tolerated, and more activity should help but may not be enough. At this point, stool softeners or laxatives may be needed; ask the health care provider for specific advice.

Diarrhea

There are also many difficulties on the other end of the spectrum. With diarrhea, frequent loose stools or the inability to control bowel movements can be a major lifestyle-limiting situation. Here, too, the elder should undergo a medical evaluation to see if there is a fixable problem. After these possibilities have been explored and ruled out, the only option may be to simply manage the problems, focusing on adequate hydration and cleanliness.

Pain

In advanced age, pain is ubiquitous. Everything has the capacity to hurt: heart, head, belly, joints, muscles, fingers, and toes. These problems are as old as old. Pain can be localized or everywhere. It can be constant or intermittent, dull or sharp; the descriptions are endless. Causes can be clearly identified or mysterious and inexplicable. The treatment of pain can be straightforward or complex. The effects of pain and the side effects of treating pain may limit functional status in major ways. The ability to sleep, get out of bed, move through the day, eat, and enjoy life are just some of the things affected by pain.

Pain is considered to be "anything the patient says it is," and therefore is a totally subjective experience. There is no test or objective way to quantify pain, but there are some standard tools used to help keep track of the patient's experience and response to pain. The ten-point rating scale is often used, with 0 indicating no pain at all, and 10 representing the worst imaginable pain. There are also the diagrammatic representational scales of smiling and grimacing faces. Also useful are the ancient one's own descriptions of the pain, particularly word choices such as *sharp, burning,* or *aching.*

Nonverbal manifestations of pain are very useful indicators of overall comfort status. Facial grimacing, wincing, moaning, increased pulse, blood pressure, sweating, squirming or unusual stillness, and/or guarding or protecting a particular body part can serve as bigger clues than what is actually said about what is going on.

Cognitive impairment complicates the assessment of pain, and the caregivers may need to rely upon these nonverbal cues. Often pain provokes behavioral disturbances in those suffering from dementia, and good pain management can improve overall cooperation, appetite, mobility, and sleep. However, these are the same folks who can experience sedation or increased confusion with strong pain meds, so caution is advised.

Acute pain from an injury or surgery needs to be managed while maintaining a balance of alertness, comfort, and function. This pain may be severe and require strong medication. These meds may be effective but carry a lot of risk in the elderly. Mobilization, getting the person up and moving, is very important for recovery. This recovery is often slowed down by pain or by the lethargy, confusion, dizziness, or nausea that comes with pain meds. These complications have the potential to overshadow and outlast the pain that started it all.

The first step of chronic pain management is trying to avoid the precipitants of pain. If movement is the thing that causes pain, activity may be curtailed. However, this may in fact result in progressive weakness. This is a trend that just causes more trouble. Our ancient ones need a balanced approach with an activity or exercise program to maintain strength. Sensible modification of the normal routine may mean using a wheelchair for long distances or limiting the number of times a day that is spent climbing stairs. When pain is a factor, adaptive equipment for activities of daily living (ADLs) or more household or personal care should be considered.

Pain meds are numerous and come in many forms, including liquids, pills, injections, and skin patches. It's important to note that over-the-counter options, such as anti-inflammatory meds and acetaminophen, can cause stomach problems—from irritation to ulcers—and are hard on the kidneys and liver. Narcotics are strong pain relievers with a wide range of dosing options; these have the side effects of sedation, confusion, and constipation, all of which can be serious problems.

Pain can come from disease or disorders in body systems, such as heart disease or stomach problems. These problems are treated with medications that aim at the source of pain. Other types of medications that can be prescribed to manage atypical pain include antidepressants and anticonvulsants. This is often a trial-and-error approach to these difficult problems, and patients should make sure to give their physicians honest feedback, using the pain scales, so adjustments can be made as needed.

The following story is an example of the trade-offs that may occur when pain treatment must be balanced with other mental and physical issues.

Lucy

Lucy was ninety-five and in relatively good health when she fell and broke her hip. Her surgery was uneventful, and she did well—until she woke up. At that point, she was confused and in pain. The pain meds, although necessary, both sedated and confused her. She ate and drank insufficient amounts and was mildly dehydrated and had low blood pressure. Because she was drowsy when she ate and drank, she aspirated and developed pneumonia. This set off her chronic lung disease, and the medicine for that problem caused restlessness. Then she retained fluid and developed congestive heart failure. It took a great deal of effort to find the right balance to sort all of these issues out effectively, but eventually Lucy was well enough to go to rehab and start the recovery process.

Pain clinics and palliative care programs are evidence that the healthcare community is using new approaches to address the serious and debilitating effects from chronic pain. From joint injections to complementary therapies such as acupuncture and massage, there is more to pain relief than just medication. Whenever pain is an issue, be sure to explore several different avenues of potential relief.

Chapter Eight

Care Where?

Depending on the elder's condition and available levels of support, treatment may occur in a range of places, from the home at one end of the spectrum to a nursing or hospice facility at the other. This chapter looks at all of these options in more detail to help you make the best choices and ensure that ancient ones receive the care and support they need.

At-Home Care

In many cases, the time comes when an elder needs some form of ongoing assistance to be able to live at home. For instance, when an elder needs personal care, the family needs to make additional plans. I have seen countless variations on the plan, from family members who quit their job and relocate in order to serve as the personal attendant, to those who move the elder into an already crowded dining room at their own residence or fit in several drop-by visits each day. Each time, I am struck by the magnitude of their effort. This work is not easy, and millions of people are doing it every day in one capacity or another.

To help make home-care possible, many people use a combination of the informal assistance from family and friends and the formal services provided by a variety of agencies. Other families choose to have all of the elder's home care provided by the formal care programs from nursing agencies, community elder agencies, or individually hired attendants.

Elder care agencies are a vital part of our healthcare system. These services come in many shapes and sizes, and specifics depend on the location and the community resources. Options are usually either community-based programs (for those people who still get out) or home services for the housebound. Many communities have services such as

- senior centers (recreational-based social programs that may provide meals);

- adult day care (therapeutic and supervised activity-based programs);

- elderly housing (apartment buildings with variable level of support); and

- adult foster care (family-style living matching those who can provide a home with those who are in need of support).

The homebound individual may need personal care, housekeeping, financial management, food preparation, and transportation to appointments. As noted earlier, Meals On Wheels is a national program that prepares and delivers nutritious meals. Depending on the elder's location, it may also be possible to sign up for grocery shopping and delivery services, or even restaurant meal deliveries. Two-day delivery services such as Amazon Prime can offer a way for distant family members to get a wide range of items to elders within a short time-span.

To find these types of services in your community, look online or in the phonebook under "elder affairs" or "senior services." A doctor who cares for elderly patients should also be familiar with the local available services and can serve as a good resource.

Some agencies provide what is considered *skilled home care*. Often paid for by insurance, skilled home care is authorized by a physician and includes nursing and rehab services for episodic problems. Typically these are short-term services for transitioning back to home after an illness, performing wound care, and managing medications and symptoms. The prototype for this care is the Visiting Nurse Association, a national organization that provides a wide range of in-home services to support independent living.

Long-term custodial care or basic assistance with activities of daily living (ADL) may be needed for those with ongoing needs. Different agencies will set up services based on need, often with sliding-scale fees, subsidized by governmental funds. Agencies that offer services for long-term care are likely to have programs for personal care, housekeeping, shopping, and transportation. Many new and innovative programs are being developed to keep frail elders at home longer. These services are ideal for those who are limited by strength, endurance, or mobility but can manage independently for a few hours at a time.

A home care agency can provide ongoing routine care called *custodial care*. These private-pay services try to be flexible in meeting the needs of individual patients and families. Most agencies have a licensed nurse as a care coordinator who monitors care. Direct care, which usually involves assistance with activities of daily living (ADLs), is then provided by home health aides. One big benefit of working with an agency is the guarantee of coverage.

Other times an elderly person needs more of a companionship type of role, especially if mere supervision is required. This level of care can be provided by an equally elderly person such as a spouse, friend, or paid companion. These people can offer reminders to eat, take a pill, or go to the bathroom. More complicated care, such as symptom-assessment and medication administration, may require a licensed nurse to actually be present.

Personalized care plans accommodate for specific needs. For example, some ancient ones may just need intervals of help, such as getting up, going to bed, or dealing with mealtimes. Others need twenty-four-hour care, because the elders may not be left alone at all. In either case, family members may be available to provide some of the care while hiring others to fill in the gaps.

As noted earlier, one alternative to hiring a nursing agency for the organization and coordination of care is a type of "a la carte" plan, whereby the ancient one—or usually the family—tries to piece and patch together a team of workers. This may include shifts handled by family members. In this situation, the family may not require a provider with licenses or certification, and duties can be tailored to specific individual needs. This type of plan is often less expensive, but the quality and reliability of the workers can be variable. There is less assurance of coverage of shifts in the event of holidays, vacations, and unanticipated absences. These problems may be manageable if there is a local family member on hand to supervise the overall situation and fill in the gaps, but it can be prohibitively difficult to manage if this care is being directed from afar.

Obviously, sufficient financial means can be a huge advantage in these healthcare dilemmas. Those with enough money and /or long-term care insurance can usually get the home care they need. Unfortunately, many people are unable to afford this type of care and are forced to make do with the resources at hand. People fortunate enough to have family or friends to help out will manage better at home and usually for longer.

Assisted Living Facilities

Assisted living situations exist in many structures, but the general philosophy is that the elders who reside there have some level of independence. These programs usually offer assistance with housekeeping and some meal preparation. There is a lot of variability among these places with regard to personal care assistance, medication management, and the facility's willingness and ability to adapt to the resident's changing status. Some have specialty units for the memory-impaired that provide extra supervision; others require their residents to be mobile, continent (or able to independently manage their own incontinence), and able to tidy their own rooms. After an acute illness, residents of assisted living facilities often need to stay in a rehabilitation facility. It is important to shop around for a big decision like placement in an assisted living facility and know exactly what assistance is provided.

Life Care Housing Options

Life care housing options include a community-style setting with a combination of some or all of the following facilities available for residents: independent apartments, assisted living, skilled nursing, and custodial care. Life care housing options provide a mixed-care environment that offers a range of services depending on the ancient one's needs. This situation can be ideal for couples of differing needs because they may live together but receive different levels of service. The different levels of care may also help the ancient ones to stay in a single location during their eventual decline, because they can simply change floors or units to receive more advanced levels of care.

Inpatient Facilities

When an illness or other setback is serious enough that the ancient one cannot be treated at home, the care team must form a new plan. One of the first questions is always, "Where will this next step occur?" A basic principle of how and where healthcare is delivered is referred to as *level of care.* Specific criteria have been set for site-specific care. For instance, the criteria determines whether a patient needs to be in the ICU or on the regular hospital floor, and it determines whether a patient needs to remain in the hospital or can be transferred to a skilled nursing facility. Note that trends in healthcare with emphasis on cost containment can also influence where care will occur.

HOSPITALS

Hospitals are the basic healthcare institution. This is where much of the intensive work is done in medicine. Hospitals usually have emergency departments for initial evaluation and stabilization. Patients can be admitted to the hospital for evaluation and treatment of illness or injury, based on the severity of symptoms and the ability of the patient to manage the situation at home.

With that in mind, much evaluation of problems can happen at the outpatient level, where a person does not spend the night at the hospital but has tests or treatment during the day and returns home afterward. Gone are the days when someone could be admitted for the ease of treatment, when a "doctor's order" was all that was needed.

Community Hospitals

Community hospitals provide basic care for their local community. These institutions have been changing with changing times. Traditionally the norm was to have the family doctor in charge of the hospital stay. Now the elder's care is more likely to be managed by a *hospitalist* (MD, PA, or NP), who will oversee the medical care and coordinate with specialists. Hospitalists are usually hospital employees who spend all of their shifts in the hospital, rather than also trying to juggle an office practice.

All things considered, it can still be of great benefit for ancient ones to be cared for in the place where their medical history has been kept on record. Most community hospitals can treat a great variety of common (and many serious) illnesses. Local hospitals also make it more convenient for friends and families to stay involved, which is a particular benefit to the hospitalized ancient ones.

Major Medical Centers

Community hospitals do not usually have access to all the medical specialties and all the most modern treatments, and for this reason patients may be transferred to a bigger hospital. The *major medical center* is a more sophisticated facility where specialized treatments occur. These hospitals often serve as teaching institutions, where any number of specialists, subspecialists, medical residents, interns, and students can be involved in the patient's care. This is where the most up-to-the-minute treatments are usually available for any problem. This is generally not where the elder should go if the goals of care are mostly focused on comfort.

These hospitals are divided into specialized units, such as cardiac, orthopedic, medical or surgical, and intensive care. The bigger the hospital, the more specific the unit: cardiac, thoracic surgical, neurosurgical, or geriatric psychiatry.

Some ancient ones feel much more comfortable in this setting, and they deliberately choose physicians who directly admit there. As noted, others, due to escalating problems or the fact that needed treatments are not available locally, end up there after a transfer from a community hospital.

Rehabilitation Hospitals

Rehabilitation hospitals are institutions that may have outpatient and inpatient care for intensive therapy for a multitude of problems. Patients suffering from traumatic injury, neurological issues, orthopedic challenges, and other medical problems (e.g., injuries from car accidents, strokes, broken bones, and replaced joints) are treated here. These facilities will screen the potential patients to see if they are appropriate for admission. For elders to be accepted, the facility's staff must feel that the patient will be able to benefit from and tolerate several hours of physical, occupational, and/or speech therapy a day.

Very old and frail persons are often not appropriate for this setting due to the intensity of the programs. Many of the same conditions can be successfully treated in the less aggressive setting of a skilled nursing facility (SNF), which is discussed in more detail below.

Hospice Houses

Hospice houses are free-standing facilities designed to care for people in the last days of their lives. A person may choose to go there after a catastrophic diagnosis with very short life expectancy or may transfer there after a period of home hospice care when the situation is unmanageable. The goal of care at the hospice house is to provide comfort measures to the patient and support to the family in a pleasant environment. It is not a place to stay for weeks at a time, and in some cases the patient may rally, stabilize, and need to transfer elsewhere, such as a skilled nursing facility.

SKILLED NURSING FACILITIES (NURSING AND REHABILITATION CENTERS)

Skilled nursing facilities (*SNF,* pronounced *sniff*) are also called *nursing homes*. Here there is physician supervision and twenty-four-hour nursing care. There are usually on-site rehabilitation services. Medicare and other insurance pays for skilled care in this setting. Many patients are admitted here for short-term rehab and are later discharged home in improved condition with home care services arranged.

Elders who are admitted to a skilled nursing facility most often have had a three-night stay in the hospital and now have a "skilled need."[4] The skilled need is what justifies the admission to the SNF.

1. A *nursing skilled need* may relate to wound care, postoperative care, medication, or symptom management. Examples are IV therapy and wound care.

---

[4] Some insurance companies have lifted the "three-night stay" rule and allow a patient to go directly from home to rehab if indicated and there is a skilled need (an excellent idea by the way). The information in this section is based on the rules that exist at the time of writing, and even though they are not new rules, they are very much subject to change, due to the whole changing picture of healthcare in the United States. Specifically, the distinctions of need are based upon current Medicare guidelines, which are massive and beyond the scope of this discussion, so this material must be limited to an overview.

2. A *rehab skilled need* refers to deficits in functional mobility due to weakness, injury, or illness. In this case, there is a difference between what the elders can do and what they need to be able to do to return to their home environment.

In order for elders to qualify for this type of facility, the healthcare team must also expect that they will improve with therapy. For this type of care, Medicare and other insurance plans will pay the bill up to one hundred days while ongoing skilled need is required—that is, until the patient gets better and can go home or stops benefiting from these services and has plateaued at a level of care that does not match up with the original discharge plan (going home).

Elders in the latter situation may instead require *custodial care*, which means that they stay in the nursing home not to improve their condition but to get help with activities of daily living: getting meals, getting washed, getting dressed, and going to the bathroom. It's important to note that this type of care is not covered by routine health insurance. Instead, it is usually paid for in one of the following ways.

1. Patients use long-term care insurance to pay for it.

2. They pay for it privately, which can quickly become a financial burden for individuals and their families.

3. They initially qualify for Medicaid from a financial standpoint.

4. They start out as privately paying for care only to exhaust their funds and "spend down" to a point that they then qualify for Medicaid.

The fourth situation can be particularly traumatic for elders who had hoped to leave an inheritance for their family. Whenever possible, patients and their families should obtain good financial and legal advice far in advance to help sort out and plan for these possibilities.

There is also a stigma about nursing homes that patients and their families may need to address. Moving into a nursing home, often considered the least desired option, may seem like a failure in some ways. However, many ancients do quite well in a nursing home. Practically speaking, life just gets a lot easier. The presence of twenty-four-hour care with healthy meals, the proper administration of medications, and physical assistance allows for rest, instead of stress. A lot of pressure is relieved, and the daily lives of the ancient ones may actually stabilize at this point.

If the circumstances of illness lead from home to hospital to skilled nursing facility, there may be an opportunity for elders to transition from short-term rehab to long-term care in the same building. The time in the rehab portion will allow the ancient one to "try on" the place and give everyone time to see how responsive the patient is to the environment as well as how responsive the staff is to the elder's needs.

The decision to place a family member in a nursing home is generally not made recklessly or without deliberation. Nursing homes are often a person's option of last resort, and families and decision-makers often put great effort into trying to avoid this. However, the right fit can make all the difference between a negative experience and a positive one. I have seen sad, frail, and lonely people resist staying at a nursing facility for long-term care only to adjust to their new life, make friends, learn new things, and basically have a good time with an improved quality of life.

FINDING A GOOD FACILITY

Finding a good place is a question of availability, location, staffing patterns, and referrals from friends and professionals. This section provides a brief overview of what to look for as you choose a facility.

Let's say it's clear that your mom needs long-term care. Her progressive dementia makes her prone to wandering, and a recent bout of pneumonia has left her weak and prone to falls. She has a host of other troubles, including diabetes, that often require around-the-clock care. How do you pick the right place?

To begin, consider the general area where you'd like her to be. If you or family members hope to visit often, then you will want her in a facility that is close to you. To help you find a good one, ask multiple sources: her doctor, your friends, and the senior agencies in town. Call or stop by for a tour. (Unannounced visits in particular will give you some idea of what the place is like when they don't have time to prepare for your inspection.) Look for a clean, pleasant-smelling facility, and check out the atmosphere by observing staff-patient interactions. Ask yourself the following questions.

- Do residents (and staff) look happy, clean, and well groomed?

- What is going on? Are the residents engaged in pleasant or fun activities? What else is there to do?

- Does the food look and smell good? Is it presented in a pleasing way?

- How long have staff members worked there? (Staff longevity is often a good sign.)

Regulatory agencies issue yearly report cards about facilities that provide some objective information about standards of care, from the temperature of the refrigerators to the number of bedsores and the number of falls. While these scores are just one snapshot of what really goes on, ask the admissions people how they scored.

A lot of what makes a good fit between a nursing home and a resident is a matter of chemistry. I have seen an individual relocate from facility to facility until one felt right.

The horror stories that make it into the media are no doubt true, but they are few and far between when you consider just how many nursing homes exist. The best way to protect ancient ones who must live in a nursing home is first to choose the right one and then to show up and visit, engage with the caregivers, and generally stay involved by participating in as many activities and decisions as possible.

Before we wrap up the chapter, let's take a quick look at George's story to see how the "where" of care can change over time and how the patient's progress will affect the options that are available.

George

George was an independent, retired bachelor living with significant heart disease. His healthcare team consisted of a PCP who coordinated his medications with a cardiologist. One night he developed chest pain and went to the emergency room, where he was evaluated and promptly admitted as an inpatient. The hospital physicians determined that he needed heart surgery. He consented to the surgery and was transferred to a major medical center, where the cardiac surgeon performed the operation.

The surgery was considered a success, but the post-op time resulted in multiple complications that required a long stay in intensive care. It was a difficult time but George eventually made it through. After a brief stay at an acute rehab hospital, he was transferred to a skilled nursing facility for further, less intense rehab. He continued with physical, occupational, and speech therapy to work on strengthening and endurance, as well as improving the quality of swallowing and the quality of overall cognition. The nurses monitored his response to meds and tended the few wounds that George had developed along the way.

The overall goal was then to get George back to independent living. The team hoped he would progress to the point where he could return home or move into an assisted living facility. There were at least two ways this could go. If the plan was successful, then George would still require extensive home care in either location (home or assisted living), including nursing, therapy, and a home health aide and homemaker to help with personal care and housework. Meals on Wheels would be required, as well as an emergency call button such as Lifeline. Alternately, if George could not recover to the point where he could return home or to assisted living, he would need to stay on in the facility as a custodial care long-term resident, where he could receive twenty-four-hour care for any residual cognitive and functional deficits.

Based on the elder's health, which will vary as time goes on, it's essential to choose the most beneficial place and type of care. While at-home care is usually considered the ideal—and most elders long to stay at home—with the right match even a skilled nursing facility can be a great way to keep ancient ones happy, comfortable, and safe.

Chapter Nine

Mental Health

Mental health and mental illness are difficult topics to define at any age, due to the vast range of human experiences and behaviors. As well, subjectivity is always an issue. Behaviors are always evaluated in the context of the appraisers' expectations: the ways that evaluators think someone should behave or respond to a particular situation. Advanced age is not a time where this gets any easier. Our society has set some specific expectations about aging behavior, and deviation can be seen as pathology. Yet qualities such as forgetfulness, apathy, and stubbornness are common among the ancient ones and can exist in a continuum of behaviors that involve both mental health and mental illness.

The story of Beth is an illustration of several aspects of mental illness in one person. As time progressed, specific symptoms would rise to the surface and become prominent temporarily only to be replaced by the next manifestation of her illness.

Beth

Beth was a ninety-year-old woman who was a resident of the nursing home for about five years. She had been widowed long ago and had no children or close family. Her anxiety disorder was longstanding, and she had some experience with mental institutions. This explained her unrelenting fear of being "doped," and she flatly refused psych medication.

Originally, Beth had moved into the nursing home after a series of hospitalizations and rehab stays for chest and abdominal pains both thought to be from anxiety. She was a classic self-described "nervous wreck." Although she initially resisted moving in permanently, once she did, the safe supportive environment agreed with her and she was very happy. For years she had no more pain and only occasional anxiety. She was functional as well as creative, a high-volume producer of holiday-specific crocheted decorations. She showered the staff with these hand-crafted treasures. These activities kept her feeling inventive and useful, and in general her spirits were good.

As time progressed, a traumatic event from her youth began to haunt her.

The staff was never sure if the event had disrupted her entire life as much as it disrupted her last months, and they did not know what had triggered the recurrence of her mental illness, but suddenly she was much worse. Did she see something in the news or someone who reminded her of her past?

Beth started to experience more intense anxiety flare-ups with paranoia. She developed persistent and progressive feelings of persecution from the staff. She had two focuses of delusion: mainly, she was sure that (a) she had a contagious disease and the staff members were punishing her with bad and inappropriate food, and (b) they were conspiring to evict her. During her phases of food paranoia she would restrict her own food intake, and the staff simply hoped for the mood to pass so she would eat again. When she was worried about eviction, she ate more easily. Although these symptoms and behaviors were cyclical and would shift as suddenly as they came, it became clear over time that she was getting worse. She was losing weight in spite of all the efforts on the part of the staff to reassure her about her food.

The medical team tried to convince Beth that her thoughts were hurting her, and they recommended medicines to help her feel more at ease. Beth's "father knows best" attitude toward her health care should have helped in this regard, but in her case the "father" whose advice she thought she should still follow was actually a doctor who had treated her decades ago. She had a perceived intolerance to many medications and would resist most suggestions to take them. She often resisted non-pharmacological interventions as well.

Next she developed a multitude of complaints, including the original chest and belly pains, nausea, and dizziness. A number of noninvasive tests were run but found nothing. At one point she reported a pain in her arm and chest and was sent to the ER, but again nothing showed up in the tests. However, a day or so later she developed a rash, and it became clear that she had shingles, which explained her pain. Yet instead of feeling validated, she became more distressed. The standard sign on the door alerting visitors to her infection tripped her fear of being contagious. She took to her bed, both refusing care and food.

Beth's deep fear of psych medications and fear of eviction made a psychiatric admission a very unappealing option; staff members had repeatedly reassured her that she would not be evicted and strongly felt a need to continue to care for her at the nursing home. Her physical misery escalated to the point of screaming at even a light touch, and she refused most of her meals and medications, although she soon became so tortured by her circumstances that she allowed the addition of a "nerve pill." Because she wasn't eating, she rapidly lost weight and strength.

She finally consented to pain medication and something for her anxiety. The more her anxiety could be controlled, the more she could eat and the better she felt. She allowed the staff to bathe her and wash her hair. She even slept almost through the night. And she improved just in time to crochet some candy cane pins.

Common mental health problems in the elderly include depression, anxiety, and psychosis. *Delirium*, which involves disorientation, sleep-wake disturbances, lethargy, and agitation, is a potentially devastating complication, as frightening as it is mysterious. These problems are often combined with each other and coexist with medical illness and dementia. As Beth's story shows, their symptoms can present problems that seriously threaten survival.

Most medical health practitioners are usually well suited to care for fairly straightforward anxiety or depression, mild psychosis, and insomnia. More complicated or persistent problems, such as schizophrenia, profound depression, and severe anxiety, may be best dealt with by psychiatric specialists. Rarely do these conditions exist as discreet entities; rather, they often occur in combinations, such as anxiety and depression, or psychosis and depression.

A common response to mental illness in all ages is to self-medicate with substances such as alcohol, caffeine, or nicotine, or to misuse prescription medications. In those of advanced age, this often results in counterproductive side effects. Monitoring the use of these substances can provide clues to what is occurring medically. For example, the elders might be increasing their alcohol use to reduce physical or emotional pain. Yet reducing the use of these substances can actually help improve symptoms. Avoiding caffeine, for example, can lessen the severity of anxiety and/or insomnia. Decreasing alcohol use can improve mental clarity and physical functioning.

Families and caregivers who are dealing with the mental illness symptoms of ancient ones may find that religious beliefs and spiritual practices can be used to help elders through difficult times. Requesting visits from chaplains, ministers, or priests can help reorient a depressed or anxious person to their faith and promote calm. It may be possible to use their belief system as an intervention by speaking with them about it, saying prayers together, and/ or playing hymns or other religious recordings. Meditation and guided imagery may also be effective in decreasing anxiety and improving mood.

While it is one thing to have a brief encounter with an elder who struggles with mental health issues, whether to make an assessment or to provide medication to a symptomatic patient, it is quite another to be the one providing the direct and ongoing care. The days spent with an ancient one who is experiencing any combination of these problems can be very long and challenging. The attitude and approach of the caregivers can have a major effect on the course of the daily events. Rushing the patient and trying to maintain the caregiver's timeline and/or agenda may not prove to be a successful plan. A calm, nonconfrontational, and unhurried manner will often get better results than too much bossing.

Common Mental Health Problems

What follows is an overview of common mental health problems and a discussion of their effects, including suggestions for how they can be managed in the lives of the very old.

INSOMNIA

I have included sleep in this chapter on mental health because the absence of sufficient sleep overlaps with the other issues discussed in this section. Just like bathroom habits, sleep is a regular—often ritualized—event that can get out of whack for many reasons and can have serious consequences.

Sleep habits change over one's lifetime, yet the need for eight hours continues. Many elderly people feel they do not get sufficient sleep. First of all they are tired, really tired, and at this age, there just isn't enough sleep to fix that. Many physical maladies also interfere with sleep. Here are some common complaints that ancient ones may experience.

- Old bodies are stiff and sore, which interferes with sleep.

- Bladders are faulty. Elders may need to get up frequently to pee or suffer through some wetness.

- Elders who suffer from stomach reflux or those with heart or lung problems may wake in the night with shortness of breath or chest discomfort. In this case, sleeping with extra pillows may help prevent these symptoms.

It is important to find out the details of a "can't sleep" complaint. Insomnia can be due to the problem of falling asleep, staying asleep, or just waking up too early. Interrupted sleep due to physical symptoms can often be improved with treatment. Fretting or staying awake with worry is another common sleep disruptor; this is often a harder problem to solve.

There are a variety of sleep aides available, and they are heavily marketed in popular press. That does not mean they are a good choice for this frail population. In particular, sleeping pills are hazardous options for a frail and/or unsteady person. Side effects include falls that occur from dizziness, drops in blood pressure, unsteadiness, disequilibrium, or confusion. In fact, a person over eighty-five is much more likely to have an adverse effect from a sleeping pill than a good night's sleep. Other medications—namely pain medication, antihistamines, and some antidepressants—can have sleepiness as a side effect, and these options as a treatment for insomnia may be safer. A doctor should always be consulted.

It is important to note that over-the-counter medicines are not particularly safer than prescription sleep aides. Often there is also a hangover effect from these sleep-inducing meds as the aging organs lose their ability to promptly eliminate the drugs from the body.

There are many behavioral interventions to improve sleep. Here are a few things that ancient ones can try.

- Minimize caffeine and limit consumption to the hours before noon.

- Limit fluids several hours before bed to decrease the need to get up as often during the night.

- Exercise regularly to promote better sleep.

- Expose the skin to sunlight, either by going outside or sitting in a sunny window, which can help with daily body rhythms.

- Keep the bedroom dark but ensure that there is some kind of lit pathway to the toilet.

- Provide a comfortable sleeping surface with an updated mattress or pad. Just because the person is ancient, there is no reason for the mattress to be!

- Try to limit napping to thirty minutes, and complete napping eight hours before bedtime.

Sufficient sleep is crucial for a number of reasons. Ancient ones who suffer from lack of sleep develop a decreased resistance to illness and an increased risk of falls or other accidents. As well, with chronic poor sleep they may develop mental status changes such as increased agitation, and anxiety and irritability can ensue. Acute sleep deprivation that occurs in a hospital or other institutional setting can prompt a full-blown delirium, as described on page 171.

DEPRESSION

Depression is a common mood disorder traditionally defined as a pathologic and persistent sense of sadness, despair, and hopelessness. In the elderly, it can cause lack of appetite and poor sleep habits, which in turn can result in debilitation and weakness. A depressed older person easily gets run down, experiences weight loss, and becomes prone to illness and accidents. Apathy can keep ancient ones from getting exercise and participating in their favorite activities.

As symptoms persist, a treatable depression can often mimic—or coexist with—dementia. Feelings of sadness, despair, and hopelessness can make it hard for elders to seek help and report these problems. With advanced age, there are so many losses—health challenges, deaths of friends and family members, the diminishment of independence and mobility—it is, in fact, natural to have feelings of sadness. But when the symptoms interfere with functional performance, then it's time to worry.

Elders without depression can experience feelings of sadness but still maintain the desire and willingness to get out of bed to eat breakfast; patients with depression lose that desire and capability. Fortunately, with treatments such as antidepressants, many elders who suffer from depression can experience improvements in their mood and once again participate in pleasurable activities, including eating.

Without treatment, ancient ones may struggle with a depression that's severe enough to put their survival at great risk. They may demonstrate a profound disinterest in life; some may even develop a passive suicide plan and stop eating. Potential for suicide exists in this population, and it is common for people to make worrisome comments. Some comments seem to involve active plans for death, such as "If I had a gun, I'd just shoot myself!" or "Don't you have a pill you can give me?" or "I feel like jumping out the window!" Other comments are more passive, including "I just wish I wouldn't wake up!" or "I pray to God every night to take me." Some of this is just talk, drama, or figures of speech; other comments, and the way they are delivered, indicate that the elders are completely serious. Comments like these all merit investigation to identify if there is a plan or significant risk for self-harm.

Psychiatric consultation is indicated for elders with worrisome suicidal ideation. Minimizing risk may also involve reducing opportunity, such as limiting alcohol (both to minimize interactions with medications and to prevent impulsivity), and supervision of sharp objects, such as knives or scissors. Close monitoring of medication, in this case, should also be done to prevent hoarding of pills for purpose of overdose. Using a pillbox can prevent access to the contents to a whole bottle of meds.

Sometimes patients with early dementia and slow onset depression may have what was formerly called the *dwindles*. This is now called *failure to thrive*. This is a nonspecific global decline in an elderly person, not explained by another specific condition. This can present as a slow disengagement from the world, without distress or discomfort.

As with depression in all ages, physical activity can help mood, and exercise can improve symptoms. With that in mind, maintaining health habits such as proper diet, activity, and sleep can be very challenging during times of depression, and medical guidance and intervention should be sought as needed.

ANXIETY

Anxiety is extremely prevalent among the elderly, and it varies in its severity. The possibilities range from concern, to worry and anxiety, to agitation and panic. Elders have plenty of reasons to worry. They worry about their families, their finances, their health, and their pets. They often need help sorting through these concerns and setting up a plan for their resolution (if that is possible).

Sometimes the problem itself is not the issue, but rather the anxiety about the problem. In many cases, family members, friends, and other caregivers can manage an elder's mild form of anxiety with a simple behavioral plan and creative problem-solving. For instance, things like delegating duties and offering reassurance can help decrease anxiety.

Exposure to media can have a negative effect upon the elder's sense of calm. Another tragic school shooting, bloody battle, new disease, life-threatening storm, or natural disaster can prompt escalating anxiety. Sometimes all that is needed is for the elder or the family to change the radio or television station. Put on *I Love Lucy* or an old movie. When anxiety is an issue, use television and other media only for a favorable effect—laughter if possible—and skip the news.

Other forms of anxiety may be more of a challenge to address. For instance, it's also important to note that anxiety can easily escalate in the presence of physical pain or difficulty breathing. In these cases, the treatment of the physical problem, better pain management, or improved respiratory symptoms may lessen the anxiety. However, if these treatments make no impact, or if the situation is severe enough to limit sleep, diminish functional capabilities, or exacerbate other medical problems, then specific anxiety medication may be in order.

Unfortunately, many medications for the treatment of anxiety can cause dizziness, weakness, sleepiness, unsteady walking, and confusion, all of which increase the risk for falling. Anti-anxiety medications are in the same class as some sleeping pills and muscle relaxers. Some ancient ones have a long history with their use and have either a tolerance to or dependency upon them. The suggestion to limit or stop these meds is often not a well-received idea.

Anxiety can also arise as a side effect to other medications. Some respiratory inhaled meds are known for making people jittery, and oral steroids can cause mood swings. Paying attention to the timing of symptoms can help identify trends so that treatments can be adjusted accordingly.

Counseling or psychotherapy may be used for these issues and can be helpful in managing these common problems and symptoms. The availability of specialized geriatric mental health services varies with location. I encourage the use of these services for many of my patients during times of big transitions, such as loss of independence, a new reliance on personal care providers, or the need to move in for long-term care.

However, when hearing is severely diminished and/or memory is very impaired, the effectiveness is limited.

PSYCHOSIS

Psychosis is a more severe problem than depression and anxiety because it is further outside of "normal" behavior. Psychosis involves (but is not limited to) the following symptoms:

- hallucinations, which may be auditory, visual or tactile;

- paranoia, suspiciousness, or fear;

- delusions of persecution, grandeur, or youth; and

- behavioral disturbances, such as combativeness or biting or pinching caregivers.

Some elderly people have a personal history of schizophrenia and have dealt with these issues over their lifetime. Other times these symptoms can develop fairly suddenly or evolve and escalate over time.

These symptoms are hard to deal with, can be very difficult to manage, and, in some instances, are actually dangerous for ancients ones and bystanders alike. These symptoms often make life very unpredictable, and patients can quickly turn on previously trusted family members. Agitation may progress to the point of combativeness. These problems clearly need medication remedies.

This is not the time for families or caregivers to be confrontational. There is no benefit to being anything other than calm and agreeable. Redirection is better than reorientation. Make reasonable one-step suggestions, such as "Let's go over here" (or get a snack or take a walk). Simple directions need to state what behavior is wanted, not what is NOT wanted. For instance, instructions should take the form of "Please sit down" or "Come this way" rather than "Don't get up" or "Don't go there." Maintaining safety is the highest priority.

This is definitely the time to seek medical attention, and hopefully this can be done at a time when the person is calm. As these symptoms both wax and wane as well as escalate out of control, it is important to keep in touch with health care providers about these changeable situations. An elder with psychosis is a person that may have an activated healthcare proxy and the agent may be making decisions and consenting to medications. Trials of medications can be done in the home setting and may be effective and well tolerated. Alternatively, these difficult situations can require inpatient psychiatric hospitalization. An agitated delusional person may have such severe symptoms and behavioral disturbance that there is no choice but to call 911.

DELIRIUM

Delirium is a strange occurrence that is surprisingly common. This can affect from 10 percent of the general population of over-eighty-five-year-olds and it increases with age and the presence of dementia. It can occur in up to half of hospitalized patients and up to three quarters of elderly patients in Intensive Care Units. Delirium involves an acute change in mental status, with some degree of disorientation, associated with restlessness, agitation, combativeness, sleep disturbance, and/or hallucinations. This can happen suddenly and resolve spontaneously after a brief duration. Symptoms can range from mild to severe, can go away completely, or may linger for days, weeks, or longer.

Delirium involves the manifestation of brain disorganization from acute medical illness such as infections, painful injuries, lack of sleep, relocation, or some other disruptive event. Surgery and medications—especially narcotics for pain, sleeping pills, and muscle relaxants to name a few—are notorious for producing these mental status changes. In other cases, there may be no known precipitating factor.

Unfortunately, there is no test to verify or quantify the diagnosis of delirium, although blood and urine tests can rule out other medical problems. There is no specific treatment, and no clear prognosis.

In the hospital, delirium can compromise any medical care—from simple diagnostic testing to complex procedures and intensive care. As long as the patient is in the hospital, the goal of care is the treatment of the primary medical problem for which the patient is hospitalized, and the delirium is a complication. This can mean the patient needs to be subdued with medication or even physically restrained to allow the medical treatment to continue. Hospitals have far fewer regulations about these restraints than do nursing homes and skilled nursing facilities, where the interventions are used as a last resort, if at all.

The more attentive the staff and the closer the supervision, the safer elders who are suffering from delirium will be. This is easier said than done, and routine staffing patterns may be insufficient. Yet this supervisory role is particularly challenging for family members to fill. A one-on-one caregiver—who may be provided by the facility or, at extra cost, hired by family—may be needed to ensure the ancient one's safety. In many instances, this step is well worth any additional cost and effort.

A delirious person is at risk of serious harm. It may become very difficult for ancient ones with delirium to maintain fluids and hydration. Dysphagia (difficulty swallowing) and aspiration pneumonia are common, as the elderly person cannot focus on eating and drinking. Often these patients are disinterested, or they just refuse food and fluids.

Restlessness can be severe, with ongoing attempts to get out of a bed or chair onto weak and unsteady legs. This can result in injury, from minor skin trauma to broken bones or worse. When agitation is severe, elders needs medication. Sedation may follow and can be excessive and prolonged. Normal dosing patterns of medications may be ineffective, and there may be atypical or opposite responses to medications.

It is hard to plan for next steps in these complicated situations. With the debilitating effects of the underlying condition, combined with potential untoward effects of psychoactive medications, ancient ones who are suffering from delirium are not usually benefitting from being in the hospital and may be transferred to a skilled nursing facility. Until the delirium diminishes, there may be no real possibility for recovery; caregivers are simply hoping for survival until this clears. Even if the agitation subsides and the elder's appetite and strength return, cognition may not improve.

If the medical problem has stabilized but delirium persists, then improving the mental status will be the main focus of care. This care can occur at a specialized geriatric psychiatric unit or a skilled nursing/rehab facility. Treatment is aimed at promoting comfort and maintaining nutrition and hydration while hoping for the clouds to pass. In cases such as this, it is important to follow the lead of the patient. Ancient ones in these circumstances may have disrupted wake and sleep patterns, so food, fluids, and activity must be provided when they are awake, even if that involves working with them during odd hours.

If there is still a pain component, then some form of pain relief is needed. However, steps should be taken to ensure that the ancient ones receive the smallest effective dose. As well, it should be given *before* the anticipated pain is expected to begin, such as before a therapy activity or act of personal care. Whenever possible, non-medication interventions are preferred, such as ice, heat, massage, ultrasound, or topical liniments.

As caregivers and families work with elders who suffer from delirium, careful attention to nonverbal cues can point to some yet undiscovered source of discomfort, such as constipation, rash, or skin breakdown. In these cases, usual interventions are used to minimize the distress (see Chapter 7). Close observation may also yield information about the precipitants—not just of symptoms, but also of good moments. If the ancient one shows a positive response to something like music, ice cream, or a hand massage that promotes calm or pleasure, then by all means use it. Oftentimes an attentive personal care provider such as a nurse's aide will have ideas about these simple pleasures. Don't forget to ask, and listen to them.

Sometimes episodes of acute confusion are temporary and the ancient one's mind clears. Unfortunately, symptoms may become recurrent and can be provoked by a new infection, injury, move, surgery, lack of sleep, or change in medications.

Mental status changes should always be noted, because they may be early warning signs of illness, so be on the lookout for other subtle changes such as shifts in bathroom habits and the changes discussed earlier in chapter 7. Even a delirium that seems to completely resolve should be thought of as a very worrisome event that can be a possible warning sign of future trouble. I have seen fully functional elders experience post-op delirium after an elective surgery or after an acute medical illness only to have them return a year or two later with full-blown dementia.

Persistent delirium can wax, wane, evolve, and even become chronic, coexisting as a counterpart to dementia. Even with the best of care, patients with delirium in any setting—hospital, rehab or nursing facility, even at home—may suffer falls and injury, skin breakdown, weight loss, dehydration, global decline, and eventual death.

There is nothing quite like acute delirium. It should be considered "brain failure" and can be just as abrupt as sudden heart or respiratory failure. Somehow the latter problems are easier to understand, mainly because they are able to be measured or objectively evaluated; they make more sense. In contrast, delirium is a clinical diagnosis, a problem declared by the presence of signs and symptoms. An experienced clinician can recognize delirium from across the hall.

When ancient ones experience symptoms of delirium, they are unable to make decisions or consent to medical treatment. Health care proxies need to be activated, and the health care agent needs to take on the responsibility of discussing with providers goals of care and approaches toward treatment. These can be difficult conversations, and the family may feel totally blindsided by the dramatic cognitive decline.

Again, whenever delirium is present, there is the need to focus on goals and work towards minimizing the most distressing symptoms and the risk for injury.

Treatment Plans and Interventions for Mental Health Issues

The complexity of mental health issues, unpleasant symptoms, and behavioral disturbances demonstrate the need for a variety of treatments and interventions.

TRIGGERS AND AIDES FOR SYMPTOMS

The first step in formulating an individualized treatment plan is to identify precipitants of symptoms. Careful assessments will help families and caregivers understand what things make the situation better as well as worse. As symptoms arise, pay attention to the time of day, look at the corresponding activities, and see if there is a way to structure the day to promote calm. Bathing can be a trigger for agitation for some ancient ones, while a shower may soothe others. Changing the routine may create positive effects. As noted earlier, non-medication interventions such as music and massage may be very helpful.

THE USE OF PSYCHIATRIC MEDICATIONS

With that in mind, such interventions may still not be enough to keep distressed elders safe or comfortable. It may be necessary to add medication alongside these other beneficial measures.

Psychiatric medications are a group of medications that mainly affect brain function. They include medications to treat anxiety, depression, psychosis, or insomnia. The right medication or combination can relieve these potentially devastating symptoms.

Several individual medications can have a positive effect on more than one symptom. For instance, some antidepressants can help with both depression and anxiety while others can have pain-reducing effects. Others may calm the ancient one, help organize thoughts, or improve appetite and sleep. It's important to note that antidepressants often take weeks for the desired effect, so consequently other meds that act promptly may be needed in the short term to manage the distressing symptoms of depression.

Flexibility in daily pattern is also important while the ancient ones take psych medications because their sleep-wake cycles can be disrupted. In fact, this alteration in the sleep-wake pattern is a reason many people end up in nursing homes. Caregivers should make sure proper nutrition is available whenever the elder is awake, calm, and comfortable enough to eat. The ancient one's activity levels also need to be maintained, even if the best time for the patient to walk is at three in the morning.

Dosing Ranges and Combinations

There are wide dosing ranges among individual prescriptions, as well as multiple combinations from the different classes of medications. For example, an antidepressant, an antipsychotic, and "anti-dementia" medication may all be indicated for the same person to control the symptoms of apathy, poor motivation, agitation, and paranoia occurring in the context of dementia.

Unfortunately, while healthcare providers do know much about the medications that are often required to ease the unpleasant symptoms associated with mental illness, the only clear part about the use of these drugs is that there are few clear-cut answers. The safest plan for symptoms that have not reached crisis level is usually to start with a low dose. Small doses that slowly increase over time are more likely to reach the desired effect without causing harm. However, if symptoms are sudden or severe, then healthcare providers may need to take the opposite approach—that is, starting with bigger doses and then scaling back after achieving the desired effect. This second approach should be done in a supervised setting, such as an inpatient psychiatric hospital or a skilled nursing facility. The potential danger in these cases is that the high doses of medication can result in excessive sedation or other side effects. Over-medication frequently causes lethargy and poor eating habits, both in the amount of food as well as the quality or textures tolerated. Ancient ones in these situations can be at increased risk for aspiration, dehydration, infection, hypotension, dizziness, skin breakdown, and falls.

Symptoms and Side Effects

As the chapter on dementia will show, many of the symptoms of mental illness occur simultaneously, regardless of the diagnosis. Behavioral issues such as repetitive comments, restlessness, agitation, and wandering are prevalent in dementia. Depression is often ubiquitous, particularly when ancient ones realize that their cognitive decline is ongoing. Sometimes the symptoms of dementia and depression overlap, and it can be difficult to tease out the differences. Antidepressants are often helpful in relieving some of the obstacles to quality of life. If medications can improve the sleep disturbances, poor appetite, or apathy, then functional status often improves.

There are times when the patient must have medications to control behavioral symptoms. At times, it can be difficult to pinpoint the cause of these symptoms and determine how to treat them most effectively. For instance, a demented person may be unable to communicate physical complaints or discomfort, so these physical issues may manifest as the behavioral symptom of increased agitation. Psych medications won't help treat physical issues, such as pain or constipation, so the agitation may continue even as pills are taken. In a case such as this, managing the pain or constipation may improve the mood or behavior better than any psych medication. (The challenges of behavioral disturbances in ancient ones who have dementia will be discussed further in Chapter 10.)

At times, the symptoms of the mental illness can be very similar to the side effect of the medication being used, and it can be very difficult to determine what element is causing what problem. For example, a patient may take a low dose of an antipsychotic drug to help control paranoia, agitation, or restlessness. Yet even with the medication, the symptom may continue or increase in severity. Alternately, some aspect of it may improve as others get worse. Perhaps the result is that this same person is still paranoid but now can't walk well either. In these situations, the questions become

- Is this change a bad reaction to the medication, or is the dose too low?

- Does the patient need more or less of this drug or a different medication?

- If it is a side effect, is it tolerable?

Oftentimes, the answer to these questions is, "It's hard to tell." Consider that these are very frail and vulnerable individuals at great risk in terrible situations. As I work with such patients, my primary plan—and a very real concern—is to avoid making matters worse with these medications. Inadvertently, however, psychiatric medications may cause dizziness, nausea, constipation, headaches, anxiety, or seizures.

Monitoring Treatments

Fortunately, careful observation by family and caregivers can minimize the hazards that often come with the use of psychiatric drugs. Friends and family members should watch the ancient ones closely for any behavioral, physical, and mood-related side effects and report these symptoms to healthcare providers, who can tailor the treatment to the individual's history and needs.

The long-term use of psychoactive medications will need to be continually reviewed by providers to make sure there is sufficient good effect and no bad effects—or at least that the good effects outweigh the bad effects. Medication combination and doses will often be changed to adapt to a changing patient status and response to medications.

In long-term care facilities, there are regulations with close monitoring of psychoactive medications. The "gradual dose reduction" is one such regulation that requires prescribers to consider a dose reduction of these meds every six months. It prompts efforts to ensure that the lowest effective dose of these potentially sedating medications is being used to control symptoms. This is a good idea in principle, but it is not without risk in practice. In many ways, it is like trying to fix something that isn't broken. Specifically, it is hard to tell if a well-functioning—but still impaired—elder is doing well because of the medicines, or in spite of them. With this approach, the way to find out is to decrease the dose and see what happens. When the ancient one remains well and does not experience a worsening of (or return to) symptoms, that indicates that a lower dose is effective. However, when elders with symptoms that were previously well controlled become anxious, agitated, or delusional because of the decrease in their medication, their quality of life may decline, and that quality is not always easy to reverse.

I think this is a good example of a common conundrum in health care. From the providers' point of view, we want to provide "good" care. Yet this may not be possible when we are obligated to follow external or regulating guidelines of care. In the example above, truly good care would involve ongoing evaluation of psychiatric meds, but it would not require adhering to a generalized timeline for an individualized plan of care.

Because of some of these regulations, providers are frequently forced to sacrifice the wellness that is occurring "today" with the interest of helping "tomorrow." For instance, we risk the delicate balance of today—that is, what is working well at the moment—for the comfort of knowing we are using the elusive "lowest effective dose." If the goal of symptom relief is achieved, then why are we worried about theoretical longer-term risk?

It is also true that even though a particular medication was effective, it was well tolerated, and its use was well justified in the past, it may still cause trouble in terms of adverse effect now or in the future. An important part of the medical care of these frail elders is to continually assess the need for and response to any of these treatments. As the next chapter on dementia describes, there is no stable status quo in the slippery slope of advanced age.

Chapter Ten

Sliding Away: The Process of Dementia

The cycle of life is a term that is often used to describe the seasonal changes and the passage of time. It calls to mind birth, growth, decline, and death. Dementia causes ancient ones to move into the two final stages—sometimes rapidly. With the onset of dementia, an elder who has been an independent and capable adult suddenly steps off the edge of time and place and starts sliding away.[5] The slope of cognitive decline—the arc of the curve—is subject to change, but the course is plotted. Traits that for years have made up an ancient one's identity begin to change on every level. Yet denial is a common reaction to the changes that are occurring. The denial can be on the part of the patient, the family, or even healthcare providers.

One of the most pressing concerns when dealing with a person with dementia is the changing need for supervision and assistance. Specifically, as the disease progresses, the ancient one will lose the capacity to remain independent. Personal safety is of great concern at all stages of dementia, and the strategies to minimize risk change over the course of the disease. However, inexperience with dementia, coupled with denial, can leave family members totally unprepared to deal with the decline and the fact that the patient is now at serious risk for harm.

As cognition deteriorates, it will also be necessary to activate the healthcare proxy so the agent can make decisions. Steps should be taken as early as possible to make sure that all paperwork is signed and in place. If the elder has not yet established advance directives, it is not too late (see Chapter 1). During times of lucidity, discuss medical issues on a very basic level, appoint a healthcare proxy if this has not been done, and consider the elder's wishes for or against life-sustaining options. Remember that time is of the essence because this lucidity may be quite short-lived; as the disease progresses, the intervals of mental clarity will be replaced with more and more periods of disorientation.

Any plan that involves a person with dementia needs to look ahead for disease progression and the practical aspects of expected changes. Of course, when the ancient one has a caregiver at home or nearby to provide some support, it is easier to feel confident that a safe plan is in

---

[5] For the purpose of clarity, dementia in this chapter refers to cases where the reversible types have been excluded.

place. Yet support should also be considered *for the caregivers*, who can easily reach the end of their rope. Friends, family, and healthcare providers should be aware of the strain involved in providing this type of care. Physically active individuals with dementia are a handful. They rarely sit down and seem to never stop moving. They may catnap during the day, or they may hardly close their eyes. Sleep patterns are frequently altered, and they may be up many times throughout the night. They may even sleep all day and be up all night. It's helpful for caregivers to get away, even briefly, but that means making arrangements for elder-sitting. Nursing home placement may also be considered at some point along the continuum.

Dementia can have many different causes. Behavioral problems and psych symptoms are not uncommon with any form of dementia, and regardless of cause there will be similar issues in all forms of dementia.

This chapter is intended to provide practical information about the different stages of and possible treatments for the symptoms of dementia. Family members and agents can then use this information to work together with the healthcare team to keep their loved ones as healthy, comfortable, and safe as possible.

Early Symptoms

Let's take a look at how one elderly woman experienced a typical decline that eventually led to the diagnosis of dementia, and how she progressed through her devastating disease.

Ginger

Ginger became a widow several years ago and moved to a new state to be closer to her daughter and grandchildren. She found a small apartment that was located both near her family and close to a park where she could easily take her daily walk. Things started out fine, and she seemed to settle easily into her new life. Looking back, her daughter reports that Ginger started to exhibit some strange behaviors, but at the time it was easy to explain away her oddities. For instance, she manifested some forgetfulness, but she had a lot on her mind. She got lost a few times, but she was new to the area. There were blank periods in the day that Ginger couldn't account for, but that was probably because she had been napping. There were some miscommunications, but Ginger did suffer from a mild hearing loss.

As time went by, however, her family members could no longer ignore her paranoia and intermittent disorientation. Ginger frequently called the police to report intruders; once she was sure it was a long-dead brother. Her daughter brought Ginger to the doctor. The medical workup ruled out the presence of a reversible cause of symptoms, and she was diagnosed with Alzheimer's disease.

Early symptoms of dementia can be subtle, intermittent, and easy to miss. When the decline takes a long time to develop, families tend to adjust to these subtle changes, which become the "new normal," and nobody notices anything amiss. Long-standing personality traits may help to cover up deficits. Homebodies who become less willing to venture out of the house might not prompt concern, particularly if the change occurs at the start of a stay-at-home season such as winter, and socially gracious elders may be so polite that they can converse without actually saying anything to trigger suspicion. People of high intelligence can also decline for a while before family and friends notice deficits.

At some point, however, problems do become apparent. Often, casual contacts are the ones to first notice that things are amiss; a fresh pair of eyes can see what the family has overlooked. For instance, tellers may call to report mistakes in bank accounts. Pharmacists may phone to report that medications are not being picked up or refilled on time. Friends and families should always take these reports seriously and schedule medical evaluations for the ancient ones.

Common Types of Dementia

Dementia is a devastating diagnosis. Treatment is limited and the disease is chronic, progressive, and terminal. It is never reversible. Conditions that are inaccurately described as reversible dementia, such as delirium, depression, or hypothyroid, are not actually dementia. A few of the common types of dementia will be discussed here.

ALZHEIMER'S DISEASE

Alzheimer's disease is just one of many types of dementia. Elders with Alzheimer's disease do not simply forget where they put the keys; they lose the understanding of the purpose of keys. This is a specific form of dementia that may have a long duration. Average duration between onset and death ranges from four to sixteen years. Symptoms present at a younger age than in many of the other forms of dementia. Alzheimer's also has distinct characteristics, including episodes of severe behavioral problems with agitation, paranoia, and wandering. This is a troublesome combination with relatively strong and fit people who essentially have acute psychotic episodes. These are not frail elders at this point.

Alzheimer's has some predictability in its unpredictability. With early Alzheimer's, there is a characteristic waxing and waning of mental status. Periods of confusion and disorientation often alternate with periods of lucidity. As noted, this is particularly distressing for ancient ones as they become painfully aware of the implications of the disease. The terror experienced when these elders discover that they feel lost or disoriented in a normally familiar setting is hard to fathom. Reassurance is a fine idea, but during these confused or agitated episodes, they may have little effect. The tone of interaction may be more important than the content. Not much makes sense to them during these times.

Reassurance during periods of lucidity is also a fine idea, but it will be forgotten when it is most needed. Repetition is needed, but caregivers should keep reassurance to a few simple statements. An example would be, "You are ok. We are waiting for your son. He is at work. You are ok. We are waiting for your son. He is at work." Doing this can be very tedious, but only to the caregiver; our confused friend has forgotten it already.

MULTI-INFARCT DEMENTIA

Another common type of dementia is *multi-infarct dementia*, which is caused by a series of small strokes. This type causes a stepwise decline in thinking and physical functioning. Ancient ones with this type of dementia go along at the same functional level for a period of time and then their condition deteriorates. That deterioration will then be followed by another big or small change and a new baseline. These steps vary in duration of plateau and depth of decline and may remain at the same level for any amount of time, then unpredictably change. This situation may reveal an occasional step up in functioning with intervals of improvement, but the general slope is down.

SENILE DEMENTIA

Old-fashioned *senile dementia* is marked by a gradual loss of awareness of reality, starting with short-term memory loss and progressing to simple-mindedness. For the most part, elders with senile dementia are very old and often do not exhibit a lot of troublesome behaviors. Instead, there is a slow disengagement from the world into another—often peaceful—place. Causes of senile dementia may include hardening of the arteries and lack of good oxygenation to the brain as the result of cardiac or respiratory problems. Sometimes this seems to be the result of fatigue; some of these very old people are just so very tired.

METABOLIC ENCEPHALOPATHY

The brain can be and is damaged by a variety of substances and medical problems. The broad term of *encephalopathy* means "something wrong with the brain." This can be caused by the negative cognitive and physical effects of alcohol, drugs, or kidney or liver disease.

General Concepts in Dementia Care

Dementia is characterized by the elder's inability to interpret the outside world. This is often evidenced when the ancient one withdraws from social situations and shows disinterest in the events in the world. For people with dementia, former interest in politics, sports, and community happenings fade away. Later, as the disease progresses, family members blur together and the elders can't find their way out of the kitchen.

Later still, dementia also causes the inability to process information from the world within. At that stage, the elders become unable to interpret their own body's cues. For example, the sensation in the pelvis that prompts healthy adults to go to the bathroom may instead give rise to another behavior in a demented person, such as irritability or restlessness.

In fact, agitation among ancient ones with dementia is a common response to a wide range of stimuli. Think of the challenges of trying to comfort crying babies who can't vocalize what they want, feel, or need. To stop the crying, caregivers may try to feed, burp, diaper, swaddle, play music, and/or take the baby for a car ride. Caregivers of elders with dementia experience the same sorts of challenges because the ancient ones, in this condition, are often unable to verbalize their needs. Following a familiar, regular routine can be an effective technique to minimize problems, and the ability—or inability— to follow that routine can also serve as a measure for caregivers to identify changes in the ancient ones' condition.

This section provides a brief overview of some of the general concerns that families and caregivers face as they manage the care of elders with dementia. More resources can be found in the reference section of this book.

EXERCISE AND SOCIAL ACTIVITIES

A healthy body is the best defense in the constant assault of age and debility. Elders who are facing dementia still need to maintain their physical capabilities, such as strength, balance, and endurance. They need to walk and exercise as much as possible. Dancing engages a drifting mind by connecting it to the body. Creative activities, puzzles and games, music, and conversation are important ways to stimulate the mind and sharpen cognitive skills. Encourage participation in social settings—including family gatherings, places of worship, or clubs—as long as it does not provoke agitation or put the ancient one at risk of injury, such as falls and wandering. Expect unpredictable behavior and continually assess the benefit of such activities as dementia takes its course.

ADDITIONAL HEALTH AND DENTAL ISSUES

As discussed in previous chapter, the management of medical conditions, particularly ones with uncomfortable symptoms, will affect mental status. Untreated anxiety, depression, pain, and even constipation can cause non-specific distress and worsen overall status.

The presence of dementia will complicate the evaluation of all subsequent health issues. As comprehension deteriorates, it becomes more difficult to get meaningful histories from the patient and explain medical procedures. Consent and cooperation are frequently variable and inconsistent. Dental work should also be done while the patient is still cooperative. Make medical and dental appointments in the morning if there is any hint of sundowning. If the medical appointment is to demonstrate and assess cognitive impairment, then make a later afternoon appointment so the assessment considers the full spectrum of difficulties.

HEARING AND VISION

Ancient ones who are newly diagnosed with dementia should get a good assessment of hearing and vision, if it's not already too late. Note that the chances for these accurate assessments diminish as the disease progresses. Don't put it off. For instance, a demented person needs to be able to cooperate during an eye exam in order to get the proper prescription for glasses; otherwise it is hard to tell what changes are needed.

For people with dementia, corrective devices such as glasses or hearing aids can actually present problems. For instance, hearing aids can be disorienting if not set properly, or overstimulating if the volume is set too high. Also keep in mind that both glasses and hearing aids have the habit of going missing, particularly when folks with dementia do unpredictable things like storing bifocals in the freezer. Keeping spare glasses as a backup is a good idea, but hearing aides are expensive, so try to help keep track of where they are placed.

MEDICATIONS

At the time of diagnosis, it is likely the healthcare provider may suggest a medication to slow the debilitating progression. The hope is that medication will help preserve the ancient one's functional status and delay the need for extensive personal assistance or nursing home placement. This is a fairly recent option in medicine, and there will likely be more medications available in the future. However, there are many questions associated with this type of treatment. It's difficult to judge the efficacy of a medicine with the goal of slowing the progression of an otherwise unpredictable course. As well, the patient may be too impaired to communicate possible side effects. Although statistics indicate these medications are effective, it's harder to gauge the individual's benefit.

With that in mind, since the medical profession has little else to offer to affect the course of this catastrophic disease, the possibility of slowing the progression usually seems to be worth the risks of side effects, especially at an early stage. Medications can (and should) be stopped at any time if they don't appear to be useful. Whenever a medication is added, caregivers need to be attentive and observe the elder for intended and adverse reactions.

In some cases, slowing down the progression isn't always desired. When cognition is severely impaired, functional status is poor, and distress is present daily, then dementia can become emotionally painful to the ancient ones and their loved ones. Prolonging the resultant impoverishment of body, mind, and soul may not be consistent with the elder's wishes and should not be considered the standard of care.

INPATIENT TREATMENTS AND HOSPITALIZATIONS

When people in any stage of dementia must go into inpatient care with a medical event, their ability to function independently and to cope mentally and emotionally often plummets. Coping mechanisms that kept them fairly functional at home can break down quickly in a different environment. The disruption of their routine can have a dramatic and negative impact on their behavior. Agitation, delirium, or acute paranoia can result, putting them at risk for injury, and may require medication.

In a hospital setting, patients often require medical interventions that need cooperation. Examples include IVs, special dressings, heart monitors, and other monitoring tools. However, confused patients often cannot remember why these devices are there or why they should be left alone. Others simply act out on their feelings of defiance.

In order to continue the medical care, it may be necessary for providers to employ the use of restraints such as fabric straps, which essentially tie the patient's hands to the bed frame. Restraints may also be used to keep a restless person from falling or climbing out of bed. In cases such as this, the restraints usually take the form of a kind of vest that is strapped to the bed.

Note that these physical restraints can be dangerous, and hospital staff needs to carefully supervise the individuals whenever restraints are in place. As well, the loss of freedom of movement can provoke an escalating situation of agitation.

Restraints were widely used in both the hospital setting and in nursing homes at the beginning of my career. While they are still used in hospitals, thankfully they have been regulated out of use in long-term care facilities. Alternatives to physical restraints that may work well for ancient ones include alarms that are designed to make a loud noise or musical tune if triggered by unwanted movements, such as when a person gets out of bed. There are also pressure-sensitive pad alarms, which sound as feet hit the floor.

None of these alarms are a good replacement for intense supervision. Many have false positives whereby the alarm goes off but the person is fine, which can result in frequent loud and noxious noise that causes further agitation. Another problem is that these devices alert staff only after the fact—that is, when the patient is already up rather than during the attempted movement.

The term *chemical restraint* refers to several classes of medication intended to subdue patients and includes antipsychotics and anti-anxiety medications. However, responses are unpredictable, and side effects are common with these types of drugs. While chemical restraints may look better than physical restraints, they are a different kind of risk and no less dangerous.

The Stages of Dementia

It has been my observation over the years of working with the elderly—and particularly those with dementia—that they go through many transitions that are similar (in reverse) to the stages of childhood. Just as the growing child will have predictable "firsts," there will be many "lasts" for elders, such as the last time it is safe to drive or to be left alone, or the last time it is possible to prepare a meal or recognize a loved one. Yet even though it's difficult, it's important to appreciate these ancient ones for who they are now, without being overcome by the loss of who they once were. Expectations and the plan of care need to keep up with the reality of the situation.

Another loss experienced during a dementing illness is the loss of functionality. As the disease progresses, the ancient one goes from being totally independent to being totally dependent. For that reason, the analogy of reversing the stages of a maturing child can be very useful.[6] This frame of reference for viewing functionality is familiar to families, and it is easy to understand in concrete terms.

An infant is totally dependent for all aspects of care. However, little by little, less assistance is needed, until the stage comes when parents are not really doing things as much as just supervising things. The decline associated with dementia involves the de-evolution of capacities, as elders begin to go in reverse. Caregivers go from supervising activities to actively taking over the care. It may start with giving the ancient one reminders to get dressed or to go to the bathroom and then progress to fully helping with the dressing or even the "paperwork" in the bathroom.

Framing the functional level of elders with dementia as *teen, preschooler, toddler,* and *infant* is a very relatable way to focus on current self-care strengths and weaknesses. This also clarifies the hazards and risks of lack of supervised care. The following sections provide an overview of what caregivers can expect when ancient ones enter each stage of dementia. At the end of the section, you will find an easy-to-follow chart to help you come up with suggestions to face the challenges of each stage.

THE "TEEN" STAGE: FUNCTIONAL BUT OFTEN ANGRY OR DEFIANT

To gain a better understanding of the "teen" stage of dementia, let's return to Ginger's story.

Ginger

Family members were very proactive in Ginger's care. The diagnosis, while tragic, prompted family members to try to keep Ginger as safe and as independent as her condition would allow. While she still had periods of lucidity, they took her to a lawyer to get her affairs in order, and they helped her establish a healthcare

---

[6] These analogies are not intended to be demeaning to seniors or to trivialize their situation; rather, I am using these analogies simply because they make sense and are easy to relate to.

proxy and living will. Her family monitored her medications and finances, helped her with shopping and food preparation, and called her several times a day to remind her to eat and to otherwise check up on her.

Evening and nighttime became more problematic, as Ginger's paranoia would escalate in the evening hours. They were concerned that she might wander out of the house. Although her daughter attempted to bring Ginger to live with her family, the move was unsuccessful. The happy chaos of a household with young children proved too over-stimulating, and Ginger became anxious very quickly. At one point, she slapped her six-year-old grandson. Her daughter struggled to juggle her own responsibilities as a mother with being a good caretaker for Ginger.

As part of this "teen" stage, Ginger's decline was entering one of the most difficult phases of dementia: agitation and combativeness. She was losing her comprehension of the world around her, and she was prone to deep frustration and rage.

In this stage of dementia, adults become more like teenagers. They have strong, perhaps fleeting, ideas, but they lack the capabilities and living skills to implement them successfully. They can be prone to mood swings and are frequently sulky about deficits they're not willing to admit.

Keeping an eye on the finances and housekeeping chores will give observers an idea of higher-level functions of ancient ones at this stage of dementia. When symptoms progress, bookkeeping and shopping tasks will need to be delegated. It will likely become essential to take steps to ensure that these ancient ones don't drive a car.

It is common for elders in the "teen" stage of dementia to have periods of confusion, alternating with periods of lucidity. At this stage, they may still be able to be left alone for prolonged periods of time. Physically, there is no impairment from the dementia, and they are able to manage basic self-care activities. They maintain continence and grooming abilities. With some support, they can be fairly independent.

Remember, however, that depression, paranoia, and rage are common at this point. Behaviors such as these can be hard to manage—even dangerous; it is often worthwhile to treat these symptoms with psychiatric medication (see Chapter 8).

As the dementia progresses, these adults will need more and more supervision. One of the hallmarks of dementia is unpredictability. The person who used to stay put suddenly begins to wander. With preserved strength and endurance, a confused, wandering, but otherwise healthy individual can be hard to keep up with.

Sundowning is a phenomenon that occurs in the context of dementia, and it can be one of the earliest and often most problematic symptoms. It refers to a marked change in mental status that happens in the late afternoon or evening. This is a time when delusions set in, including unshakeable beliefs that prompt agitation. During a period of sundowning, ancient ones become confused and disorganized, looking for their mother, their baby, a taxi—who knows? The police or family members may be summoned by calls from the ancient ones, who report perceived intruders or "peeping toms." Attentive and loving family members can be accused of stealing. And because some family members do financially exploit vulnerable elders, all reports of potential abuse should be explored.

It can be hard for friends and family members (and even the authorities, if involved) to determine if there is a basis to any of these accusations or claims. The best way to do so is to spend the evening with the ancient one who suffers from dementia; even the presence of another adult may not make a big difference in their perception of events, so it will likely be possible to determine what is actually going on.

When dealing with individuals in this condition, honesty may not be the best policy. During these times, ancient ones are not rational, so rational explanations will not satisfy them. Provide them with an explanation that makes sense to them, be vague, and remain calm. Redirect and distract their attention as needed. The caregiver's goal at these times is to maintain safety, provide calm, and de-escalate the situation.

THE "PRESCHOOLER" STAGE: CONTINENT BUT FORGETFUL

After the "teen" stage, ancient ones who suffer from dementia usually move down to the "preschool" stage. Let's take a look at how this backward progression manifested itself with Ginger.

Ginger

As we saw earlier, Ginger had specifically chosen an apartment near a park so she could continue to walk for pleasure. However, as she moved from the "teen" stage of dementia to the "preschool" stage, she changed from a recreational walker to an unreliable wanderer. Her family put bells on the doors and locked them for safety, but even when they accompanied her, she wanted to walk nearly nonstop, which was exhausting for all of them.

Because she was so determined, Ginger also managed to circumnavigate the family's attempts at safety. One day, in spite of their efforts to contain her movements, Ginger was found several blocks from home. She was wearing her parka in July and said that she was looking for her brother and the bus. Her family realized they could not keep her safely at home any longer. She was admitted to a long-term care facility.

Ginger's transition to nursing home life was stressful for both her and her family. She was frequently confused and often told the staff "Call my father" or "I have to get the baby" as well as the rational "Take me home, please." As she grew accustomed to her new setting she stopped saying those things, but instead she developed apathy and disinterest in previously pleasurable activities. At that point Ginger was treated for depression, and her mood improved but her cognition did not.

Like a child in preschool, Ginger could dress herself if she was not overwhelmed by the choices of clothes. If the aides put her clothing on the bed, she could put them on. She knew how to brush her teeth and go to the bathroom. She was very pleasant during the mornings, greeting each visitor to the nursing home with a smile and a hug and then serving as an escort through the building. During this time she could occupy herself with activities such as crafts, and she clearly enjoyed her photo albums. She was able to identify family members and remember some old stories. She would tell her favorites over and over.

Unfortunately, Ginger also suffered from sundowning. Each day, when afternoon came, her casual wandering would change into a frantic search for her brother, babies, or parents. She would become restless and uncomfortable, which progressed to delusions with hallucinations. She would reach for things—some visible, some not. She became intrusive and wandered into other people's rooms and took their belongings. Other residents, equally impaired, could get short-tempered with her behavior. The nursing staff would try various approaches to protect her from harm. She would walk herself ragged in spite of their encouragement to rest. During these times she would also become incontinent, and the required intrusion for hygiene further agitated her. She had a much harder time stringing words together to make coherent speech.

Fortunately, during the "preschool" stage, Ginger maintained her appetite, enjoyed her food, and gained weight steadily. Her family was pleased to know that this provided some nutritional insurance for the inevitable weight loss that would come down the road.

Ginger stayed in this phase for over a year. During this time she experienced a variety of medication adjustments to decrease her agitation, anxiety, and paranoia. Not surprisingly, this period was also punctuated by a series of mostly inconsequential falls. However, that phase ended abruptly when she fell and broke her hip. Admitted to the hospital for surgical repair, she had the expected rocky course, with pain and agitation management issues. She constantly tried to get up, so physical and chemical restraints were needed to keep her hip safely in place.

As time goes by, the person with teen-style dementia will become someone who cannot be left alone for extended lengths of time. As Ginger's example shows, ancient ones in the "preschooler" stage are still likely to be able to perform some ADLs (e.g., dressing, looking at photo albums) and maintain continence. However, short-term memory begins to be problematic, and the elders need more cues and reminders to meet basic needs. Caregivers need to ask questions such as, "Did you shower?" "Did you take your pills?" "Did you eat breakfast?" For elders still living at home, the situation gets particularly challenging when questions must include the consumption of life-saving medications, such as "Did you take your insulin?"

Lists or phone calls can serve as helpful reminders of what elders have done and need to do. At this point they can still talk and may be able to self-report problems. For example, they may be able to convey symptoms such as "My stomach hurts after I eat" or "My legs hurt after walking."

As time goes by, the verbal skills of these ancient ones decline, and short-term memory function may vanish. They may think their grown children or grandchildren are their parents or siblings. Sentences get lost mid-thought and much is left unsaid. The mind can get stuck in a rut, and there may be difficulty redirecting a conversation or thought pattern.

Repetitive questioning or demands from ancient ones at the "preschool" stage are common. (*Is my son coming? What's happening? Find my papers!*) There has been much debate among professionals about how much "reality orientation" is a good idea. Is it really helpful to remind demented people that the loved ones they are waiting for are dead? Do they really need to remember that they are old, broke, sick, and living in a nursing home? It may be kinder to give a response such as "I haven't seen your parents but I expect them soon" or "Yes, I'll call a cab when the phone is free." Yet these delay tactics don't always work. It is amazing to see ancient ones who can't remember anything of significance ask the same questions every hour and never seem to forget that—at least in their mind—they are still waiting for their parents to come pick them up. In Germany, several nursing homes have created fake bus stops for patients with Alzheimer's. They have found that patients who want to go home relax at this bus stop area, which usually includes a sign and a bench, because they feel like they are taking steps to meet their goal. Later, when the patients forget their original intentions, staff members invite them back in for a snack.[7]

THE "TODDLER" STAGE: MOBILE BUT UNSAFE

As noted, the trial of the hip repair and the hospital stay seemed to mark an end to Ginger's "preschooler" stage. Let's take a look at how this progressed into the "toddler" stage.

Ginger

After the hip repair surgery, Ginger returned to the nursing home for rehab. The hope was that she would regain her capability to walk, but it was clear that she had lost a lot of ground. No longer recognizing familiar faces, she was also losing the ability to make her needs known. Therapy was limited by her worsened cognitive status. She no longer had the ability to follow directions or return to a natural state of mobility. For example, she had forgotten how to walk and couldn't figure it out.

At this point wandering became a thing of the past. She was no longer as agitated during the day, and some of her medications were successfully reduced. She wasn't entirely calm, but her delusions had given way to a kind of indifference.

---

[7] You can hear more about this at www.radiolab.org/story/91948-the-bus-stop/

Ginger was now in a wheelchair most of the time. Sometimes she was able to help in her transfers from wheelchair to furniture; other times she needed to be lifted. She needed assistance with all ADLs except for self-feeding, which she could still do on most days. The staff was challenged by trying to prevent the problems associated with her relative immobility, including skin breakdown, contractures (the hardening of tissues, muscles, and tendons), and pneumonia.

At the "toddler" level, demented elders may still be walking around, and are sometimes able to find their room or the kitchen, but they are likely to get lost out of doors. As symptoms worsen, they may get lost in one room. Dangers lurk everywhere. Continence is not common, but caregivers who are well trained can minimize accidents by making bathroom visits part of the routine.

Behaviors can be troublesome if the ancient ones resist personal care. Their language skills decline, so simple directions are best. Food often needs to be modified to facilitate nutrition. They may have trouble chewing and need their food chopped or cut up finely. Smaller, more frequent meals or finger foods may be more suitable for those with short attention spans. Finger food is also good when they forget how to use forks. Following suit, if the food is not tasty, they will often spit it out. Oftentimes, anything resembling manners is well out the window at this stage.

It is not uncommon for demented elders to lose weight at this point. Liquid supplements or fortified milkshakes can be added to the diet if weight loss occurs or if food intake is insufficient. Caregivers may find it helpful to loosen the usual dietary restrictions, such as a previous limitation on salt, fat, or cholesterol. As noted earlier, sometimes the best food for these folks is the food they will eat. And while medications will not help with the problems of cognitive loss or swallowing, several different types—from antihistamines and antidepressants to hormones and THC (the primary psychoactive ingredient in marijuana)—can help stimulate the diet, thereby preventing weight loss.

THE "INFANT" STAGE: TOTALLY DEPENDENT

Unfortunately, there is simply no way to stop the inevitable progression of the disease. Before we conclude this discussion, let's take a look at how Ginger progressed to the "infant" stage, coming full circle with the start of her life.

Ginger

As Ginger's dementia progressed, she developed swallowing problems. She forgot how to feed herself; she needed to be fed. She would chew and chew and spit out some of her food. Some of her food also ended up in her lungs, causing respiratory infections. To try to prevent this, it was necessary to thicken the liquids and puree the solids; basically, her meals resembled baby foods. At this point, she experienced an ongoing weight loss. Even though she'd started out fairly plump, she was wasting away. At eighty-four years old, she suddenly seemed ancient. Like an infant, she began sleeping much of the day and had generalized responses to any uncomfortable symptom. She still tried to speak, but it was more like babbling. Observing for subtle changes in behavior and eating and bathroom habits, became the best way to identify problems like pain or constipation or even urinary tract infections, which she sometimes developed.

Dementia is a disease that persists, and the late stage is the infantile period. This is a different—but still difficult—time for loved ones. Ancient ones at this stage of dementia may no longer recognize family, but their behaviors are not as troublesome and they no longer wander. Instead, they stay where they are put and usually eat what they are fed. They now need total care, requiring assistance with ADLs: bathing, eliminating, dressing, and feeding. Eventually they need frequent repositioning to prevent bedsores, contractures, and pneumonia. Decline is inevitable, and these complications can occur even with the best of care.

It is often tricky to interpret symptoms, which can be subtle or generalized. A consistent, attentive care provider is the best person to pick up on subtle changes such as a slight shift in mental status, an unusual posturing, increased lethargy, or increased agitation, which can all be early signs of an impending illness. A foul odor of urine may suggest an infection or dehydration. An increase in respiratory rate can be a subtle sign of early pneumonia. Restlessness can be a manifestation of pain. Decreased appetite can be a symptom of pain, a side effect of medications, or the result of constipation. These signs can also be caused by the progression of the disease of dementia.

At the "infant" stage, ancient ones who are seemingly frail may actually survive for years. Their longevity is a testament to the good care provided at the most basic level. It is the caregivers who are feeding, positioning, and bathing these patients, thereby keeping them alive.

Dementia and debility progresses at the "infant" stage until there is an incompatibility with self-sustaining life. This is often a result of swallowing difficulties, and the only option for survival becomes a feeding tube. When considering the circle of life progression, this would have to be the fetal stage, and the tube would be comparable to the umbilical cord.

Summary and Stage Chart

The material in this chapter has focused on the typical progression of symptoms experienced by ancient ones who are suffering from dementia. Of course, no individual will follow the exact same path. Furthermore, the stages of dementia often overlap, and each individual's strengths and weaknesses will be evident. Some skills may be lost early on while others may persist longer than expected. Knowledge and preparedness for what lies ahead can help families and caregivers maintain their focus on supporting the overall goals of care, maintaining quality of life, and promoting comfort and safety.

The following chart will help you identify the specific challenges for each stage, and it will point you in the right direction as you seek strategies to face each challenge.

Stage	Challenges	Strategy
Teen	Wandering, getting lost on excursions, exiting premises at night	• Keep identification and address on elders at all times. • Prevent elders from traveling independently. • Keep elders in sight during outings. • Use alarms to halt exits at night.
	Depression and mood swings	• Talk with a physician about medications for depression. • Help the elder maintain fitness. • Offer calm activities. • Encourage supervised socialization. • Add structure to help maintain orientation.
	Safety, judgment problems	• Use lists, notes, and visual cues to serve as reminders.

Stage	Challenges	Strategy
Teen (continued)	May be alone for long stretches of time unsupervised	• Check in by phone at various times of day for med reminders and symptom monitoring. • Perform drop-in visits whenever possible to reassess the ability to stay alone. • Review the elder's ability to drive; take preventative steps as soon as they are needed.
	Needs cuing for or assistance with some high-level ADLs	• Set up home help for driving, errands, chores, and high-level ADLs. Delegate finances and medication management.
Preschooler	Wandering, exiting premises unsupervised	• Arrange for twenty-four-hour supervision.
	Safety concerns	• Apply "baby-proofing" measures. • Address any cooking or smoking concerns.
	Diminished mobility	• Create an exercise routine. • Make sure the elder is engaged in activities to keep fit.
	Mood swings, tantrums	• Arrange for psych meds as needed. • Make sure the elder avoids overstimulation, fatigue, hypoglycemia, and hunger. • Review meds for unwanted side effects.
	Communication difficulty	• Provide calm, structured environments and routines. • "Read" nonverbal cues.
	Struggles with ADLs; some issues with incontinence	• Assist with ADL cues, set-up, and supervision. • Provide toileting reminders.

Stage	Challenges	Strategy
Toddler	Inability to handle ADLs	• Provide twenty-four-hour physical assistance.
	Incontinence	• Purchase incontinent pads, pull-ups. • Schedule frequent toileting.
	Eating problems	• Alter diet as tolerated. • Provide smaller, more frequent meals. • Serve finger foods. • Support nutrition with supplements.
	Walking problems, safety concerns, and falls	• Minimize obstacles, distractions, and "trippables." • Supervise activity. • Use support equipment, such as gait belts, walkers, hip pads.
	Poor communication abilities	• Watch for nonverbal cues. • Keep language and directions simple.
	Anxiety	• Pursue medicines and non-medicine behavioral approaches. • Try redirection and distraction. • Avoid triggers. • Review meds for side effects.
	Exhausting to care for	• Arrange for caregiver support and respite.
	Struggles with ADLs	• Assist with ADL • Physical assistance may be needed.

Stage	Challenges	Strategy
Infant	Bedbound, non-ambulatory	• Provide for twenty-four-hour physical care. • Use a mechanical lift for transfers.
	Total dependency for ADLs, including feeding, hydration, and hygiene	• Feed with aspiration precautions and texture changes. • Follow up toileting/diapering with bathing. • Provide skincare and pressure relief.
	Declining skin, muscle tone, and joint integrity	• Follow basic nursing procedures. • Reposition frequently. • Support range of motion. • Protect from injury.
	Totally dependent on caregivers	• Support with medications as needed. • Use equipment that eases strain on caregiver. • Provide caregiver support and respite.

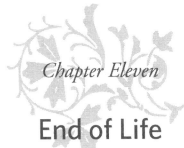

Chapter Eleven

End of Life

As our beloved ancient ones approach the end of their life, there are many physical and emotional elements to consider. Let's take a look at Sal's story, which shows some of the issues that he and his have family faced as he begins the final leg of his journey here on Earth.

Sal

Within the course of a dozen years, Sal had been admitted to a nursing facility for rehabilitation at least that many times. He suffered from congestive heart failure, chronic lung disease, atrial fibrillation, diabetes, coronary heart disease, high blood pressure, prostrate trouble, esophageal reflux, anxiety, and depression. He had survived colon and skin cancer, two knee replacements, and a broken hip.

His early admissions—after elective knee surgery and heart surgery—were quick and easy. His heart failure usually cleared up quickly. The flare-ups of emphysema took longer because the steroids gave him very high blood sugar levels, and he had skin tears that were slow to heal. When oxygen and insulin were added to his at-home plan his anxiety worsened (even though he was accustomed to these treatments in rehab), and three times he went to the ER for panic attacks he thought were heart attacks.

Sal took approximately twenty pills a day, and even more when his joints acted up. As time progressed, some of his "short-term rehab stays" got pretty long, with complication after complication. His family worked with the staff at rehab and with home-care providers to keep him safe and independent. The primary short-term goal was always for Sal to return to home. However, it was also clear that a back-up plan would be needed if that goal became impossible.

As it happens, after a particularly rocky time with persistent weakness, low blood pressure, episodes of delirium, and a few "almost falls," Sal decided to stay for long-term care. By this time he was ninety-four years old. He made the choice with the goal of trying to avoid the hospital and the ER in the future.

His family concurred that he had been to the hospital often enough to have an informed opinion and that he was tired of it.

Sal updated his Medical Orders for Life-Sustaining Treatments (MOLST) to include "do not hospitalize" and then settled into the facility, where he remains today. In fact, he is very tired, and all he wants is to be kept comfortable and to have a peaceful death. He is willing to have his usual care but nothing aggressive or heroic. At this point his episodes of respiratory distress, lethargy, and infection seem to take what little energy he has left. He rallies on occasion but he's at a whole different level now, spending most of the time in bed and eating very little. The staff has told his family, "One of these times it will be the end. He won't bounce back, and he will die." Someday it will be true.

Diminishing Returns

Getting really old takes a long time, and as frailty creeps in there are often recurrent problems—falls, infections, heart or lung flare-ups—that prompt hospitalizations and subsequent rehab stays. Commonly, patients are admitted over and over again, only to get stronger and then be discharged to home until the next time. If this were television, at first these episodes would simply look like reruns. However, as the months or years progress, the time at home shortens and the recovery time lengthens until it finally looks like the patient won't be going home again. At that point, it may be time to change the goal of care from the "rehab and homebound" plan to "supportive and custodial" care, such as a nursing home.

Even with a plan of care in place, the course of a frail elder can be rocky. There is often a cycle of decline and recovery from illness, regardless of the type of medical intervention provided (e.g., *comfort measures* versus *active treatment*). These ups and downs can be difficult to witness, prompting a questioning of previously made decisions. For instance, "ups" occur when ancient ones who are so frail and braced for decline actually improve. They may seem better at the nursing home than when they lived at home, so their families may think the elders should try again at home. But families and friends should remember that the reason for these "ups" is usually that the ancient ones are now so well cared for *in their new situations*. And then, in all likelihood, more "downs" will follow. Events such as falls, symptoms of agitation and anxiety, breathing difficulties, or simply the fluctuations of chronic illness will occur and remind everyone why the elders need to be in the new situation. It's important to recognize that these events represent the types of problems that may be fairly easily managed in a nursing home or other supervised setting but would have otherwise sent the elders straight to the ER from home, with the troubles beginning all over again.

With all of the ups and downs, it is often hard to tell whether the ancient ones are getting better or getting worse, what is a fluke and what is a real trend, how much to push for recovery, and when to back off. At this stage in their lives, ancient ones need a balance of rest and activity, and caregivers must be able to attend to their needs during all the fluctuations of their function. If the elder takes two days to rest up after even minimal exertion, such as a shower, a short walk, and visitors, then maybe better planning can spread out activities to avoid exhaustion. With gentle supportive care in place, the next step may simply be to wait and see what happens.

If the goal is care and comfort, then no more than gentle coaxing should be used to try to get the reluctant mover motivated. Staying in bed should be considered an acceptable choice for the ancient one if other preventive measures, such as good hygiene and skin care, are maintained.

It's important to note, however, that self-imposed bed rest or other limits on activity will result in a generalized deconditioning or weakening. Still, if getting out of bed or other types of movement cause pain, especially in spite of pain medications, then avoiding that type of pain is a comfort measure and the benefits outweigh the risks. Hospice care may be initiated at this point if extra support is needed.

Bedbound Care

Ancient ones will often get to the point where they decide that getting out of bed is not worth it. They are just plain tired. The simplest activity requires so much energy that they may need several hours to rest up from the exertion of it. They may be experiencing too much pain, weakness, or trouble to ever get out of bed, or they may choose to be in bed most of the time, getting out of bed only for brief intervals (ideally for meals, bathing, and toileting).

I have known frail elders who "took to their beds" and lived contently for years, so this step does not necessarily mean that the end of life is at hand. However, bed rest is a very risky activity, so—as always—it pays to look ahead at the potential consequences.

The daily (and nightly) care of a bedbound person is a basic nursing skill and very hard physical work. Depending on the size of the patient, it may be a two-person job. The basic care plan should also include maintaining the well-being of the caregivers. A traditional hospital bed is invaluable in the care of a bedbound person. It is important that the bed has the ability to be raised during physical care, to save the caregiver's back.

Professional guidance for direct caregivers is essential to manage this task. This includes tutorials from both nursing staff and therapists. Depending on circumstances, this can be done at a rehab facility before discharge or by home care agencies. Inpatient settings are expected to be capable and experienced in caring for bedbound patients.

Ancient ones who are bedridden need continual attention and assistance for feeding and cleaning, as well as for the related issues that must be addressed to minimize potential problems. These include

- skin breakdown called *decubitus*, or pressure ulcers or bedsores;

- contractures, which involve a tightening of joints in arms or legs and results in stiffness and decreased range of motion;

- pneumonia, which is the infection of one or both lungs; and

- blood clots, which can start in legs and travel to lungs.

The head of the bed should be raised to make breathing easier. Pillows can be used, but as a long-term solution they are not as stable as a bed that is designed to be raised. Eating is safest and more comfortable with the head of the bed elevated at a ninety-degree angle. Ensuring that the elder remains upright for at least thirty minutes after eating will help keep food moving in the right direction, promoting good digestion.

There is a big difference between the care of someone in bed who is able to move about in bed independently and the person who is immobile and needs to be positioned. Positioning is an important part in the care of a bedbound person. Pillows should be soft and used generously for proper positioning. They can be tucked behind the back to keep the person on one side. A pillow or two between the legs at the knees will keep proper alignment and provide pressure relief. When ancient ones lie on their back, a pillow should be placed under their calves to keep heels off the bed. Padded bed booties can help relieve pressure.

Prevention of pressure areas requires diligence. Repositioning is necessary every two hours, even during the night in the immobile person. Lotion should also be applied to bony prominences several times a day, to minimize friction. There needs to be a high-quality bed surface with smooth sheets, because even wrinkles can put the delicate skin at risk. Products such as specialized mattresses and sheepskin pads can be used to distribute weight in the bed, which decreases the elder's risk for pressure sores. (There are many high-tech products available, but some are often covered by insurance only when a wound exists.)

Keep in mind that skin is the largest organ. It can fail—evidenced by skin breakdown— just as the heart or kidneys fail when these organs lose function. Skin breakdown at bony prominences can develop in a matter of hours in the completely immobile person. The most common sites for pressure sores are the buttocks, hips, and heels, but wounds can crop up on any pressure point. Other spots vulnerable to breakdown are elbows, ankles, and ears. Incontinence is very hard on the skin, and it increases the risk for wounds.

Toileting is a challenging project with bed rest. Men can have a simpler time with urination due to the easy-to-use urinal. Bedpans are simple in theory to use, especially for urination. However, both of these devices are cumbersome and can spill.

It is much more difficult for a person to have a bowel movement in bed. If the ancient one is willing and able to get out of bed just once a day, that time should be scheduled to coincide with a bowel movement. Using the toilet or a portable commode also results in a more complete bowel evacuation, which is highly desirable since bed rest is a very constipating experience.

For the person with incontinence, it is of paramount importance to keep the skin clean and dry. Incontinent pads are often used, or the bed surface can be padded, or both, depending on individual needs and preferences. Frequent clean ups are needed and must be planned for and performed. Every two hours around the clock is advised for optimum care.

Skin and bowels are not the only things that suffer with prolonged bed rest. The musculoskeletal system also suffers with lack of use. All joints in the body should be put through their range of motion several times a day during personal care, to maintain the function of the joints and prevent painful stiffness.

Contractures or stiff flexion of joints occur with bed rest, resulting in decreased range of motion and function. This can be painful with muscle spasms. It can also be permanent and/ or progressive. Contractures frequently occur after a stroke, but they can also occur randomly, affecting one or more joints. Hips or knees can be firmly stuck in flexion, as in, curled up in fetal position, making standing difficult or sitting in a regular chair impossible.

This phenomenon also can occur in the hands, which may tend to form fists. If the elder's tendency to keep hands clenched is not kept in check, the patient will develop great difficulty opening the hands. The hands also need to be opened regularly for hygiene purposes, and particularly for nail care. The nails continue to grow throughout life and may grow into the palm of the ancient one's hand if this is not prevented.

Bones also weaken and lose mass and strength with bed rest. This increases the risk for fractures, which can occur with as little movement as sneezing, coughing, or even being turned in bed. A common occurrence is that while the ancient one is standing, the hip breaks and causes a fall. (Ordinarily, we would expect that the fall caused the hip fracture.) Any sudden pains in these very old bones are suspicious for fracture.

While problems such as bedsores and contractures are uncomfortable, unpleasant, and serious, they are not usually going to directly result in death. However, as noted earlier, prolonged bed rest also increases the risk for blood clots and pneumonia, and these can be fatal. Both of these problems are caused, in part, by the stagnation of body fluids, which truly represent how the body is slowing down. Blood clots form in the legs due to sluggish circulation, and then they travel to the lungs, where they can cause severe symptoms and death. Pneumonia occurs because of sluggish breathing, weakness with poor swallowing, and ineffective cough. At one time pneumonia was called the "old man's friend" because it was widely viewed as an illness that would carry elders to a quick and relatively painless death.

When younger patients face challenges such as blood clots and pneumonia, vigorous attempts are usually made to prevent or cure these maladies and extend life. However, at some point toward an ancient one's end or life, that strategy usually changes. Instead, these medical events are frequently expected and accepted, with the treatment approach limited to comfort measures.

Comfort Measures

Comfort measures are interventions with the exclusive goal of increasing the ancient one's comfort level. Depending on the individual's circumstance, this may require a big change in plan, such as stopping an active medical treatment plan for cancer or dialysis for end-stage kidney disease. Alternatively, this may simply indicate a subtle shift in a long downhill course. Either way, it frequently involves using medications that minimize unpleasant symptoms but may at the same time decrease alertness, mental clarity, or activity tolerance. If comfort and alertness seem mutually exclusive, then family and caregivers may conclude that options that make the ancient one comfortable but semiconscious may be more consistent in meeting the end-of-life goal than options that keep the elder alert but uncomfortable or restless.

Comfort measures also include stopping the medications that don't maintain or improve comfort. When concerns about the patient's history of illnesses or the need to decrease the risk for medical problems are removed, many meds can be discontinued. This is a philosophy of care that prioritizes the "now" far ahead of the past and the future. Blood pressure meds, anticoagulants, cholesterol pills, and vitamins are just some kinds of meds that can now be stopped.

Other interventions that may be worth stopping include physical and occupational therapy, diabetic monitoring, and dietary restrictions. Wounds that are no longer expected to heal can be treated less vigilantly if the procedures cause discomfort.

The Final Decline

The inevitability of death as the time draws near is an emotional time for everyone involved. The death-bed scenes may be played over and over in the minds of witnesses. Communication within the family and between healthcare providers is critical in providing a positive—albeit sad—experience. In the next example, the identification and implementation of clear goals allowed Lois's final decline to be effectively directed by her behavior and response to care.

Lois

Lois had enjoyed good health for most of her life. She moved into assisted living at eighty-eight years old. During the seven years she was there, she was able to see her family often and enjoyed watching her granddaughters grow up. One day, rather suddenly, she developed some confusion and shortness of breath and was whisked to the emergency room. She was found to have a "touch of pneumonia" and was admitted to the hospital. She received IV antibiotics and fluids because she was slightly dehydrated.

Next came "a little heart failure," probably as a result of the recent IV fluids, and she was treated with diuretics to drain off the excess fluid. This prompted "just a little kidney failure."

By the end of her hospital stay, Lois had become weakened from her ordeal and needed rehab to get back on her feet. Her forearms were deep purple from damage to her veins from the IV and blood draws. However, rather than getting better, she got worse.

There was no clear specific reason for her lack of recovery. A repeat x-ray showed neither pneumonia nor heart failure. Her blood work looked okay too. However, she was not taking in much food or fluids. She turned her head and said, "No, thank you."

Lois didn't refuse to get out of bed, but she wanted to go back to it within an hour of getting up. She denied pain and said she didn't feel ill. "Tired" was her only complaint.

In addition to her bruised arms, her legs had been injured in a previous fall, and the wounds were not healing. The road ahead was not catastrophic, but it looked pretty grim nonetheless. Her concerned family wanted to do the right thing by her and didn't want any futile care.

During a family meeting, her loved ones agreed that the staff should continue to offer food and fluids but not hassle her about it. Comfort would be the goal, and the staff was directed to follow Lois's lead about the direction of her care, especially as to whether or not she was interested in rehabilitation procedures. During the meeting, the staff explained to the family the natural course of likely events—specifically, the process of dying. (See section that follows.) They seemed to understand, and they prepared for her expected decline.

As her oral fluid intake diminished, Lois became weaker and less responsive. She no longer could get out of bed. The nursing staff kept her clean and comfortable, and they repositioned her every two hours. She would open her eyes from time to time, and she smiled at her son, but she was unable to speak.

Over the course of days her responsiveness decreased even more, and then it reached the point where she did not even rouse with repositioning. When she developed a fever and some labored breathing, the medical team gave her morphine drops in small but frequent doses. This helped to ease the breathing. Lois ultimately died a peaceful death surrounded by her family.

As this example shows, positive end-of-life care requires a delicate balance of support and ministrations that must be compassionate, professional, and kind. Lois's family was able to work successfully with the health care team because they were educated about the process of dying. The remainder of this chapter discusses the final stages of dying so that readers and their families will know what to expect.

The Stage of Active Dying

At some point, the slope of the elder's decline becomes steeper, and death seems closer at hand. This decline may occur suddenly and show an obvious change of status, or it may occur so imperceptibly slowly that it is hard to tell when the ancient one has entered into the active dying stage. There is no way to predict the actual timetable.

There may be a series of events that cause friends and family to brace for death, only to have the patient briefly rally. There may also be frequent dress rehearsals for "recurrent terminal decline." This phenomenon can be excruciating for family members, particularly if they have put their everyday responsibilities on hold while they support this process. For the family member who lives far away, there is the ongoing uncertainty of when to come to say goodbye.

Active dying occurs when the ancient one's level of responsiveness declines and oral intake diminishes. There will be a shift in level of consciousness, happening slowly or suddenly. Periods of alertness alternate with lethargy, and then the lethargy becomes more prominent. This phase occurs as a level of consciousness diminishes; more stimulation is required to elicit a response. At one point touch is required; in the next phase there will be no response to activities, such as personal care or repositioning. This is what is commonly described as a *coma*.

During a rally with sufficient alertness, the ancient one may still accept fluids. As long as there is a gag reflex and intact swallowing action, this is fine. Later, as the process progresses, loved ones often push fluids to meet their own needs (i.e., to do something they consider to be helpful) rather than the patient's needs (i.e., actual thirst). If choking on fluids occurs, it can help to thicken the fluids, or it may simply be necessary to accept that it is too late in the course of events for fluids. In some cases, the ancient one may tolerate ice chips in small amounts. Mouth swabs can help to moisten the lips and promote comfort.

As the dying process progresses, there are other predictable changes in the body. The respirations often become uneven. Quick shallow breaths may alternate with intervals of apnea or pauses in breathing. These pauses, which usually last about fifteen to thirty seconds, are often followed by gasps of respiration and can be unsettling to witness. These pauses may become longer and more frequent as the end is closer. Impending death is noted with the deterioration of circulation. The extremities may mottle or become cool and a dusky blue.

Vital signs (temperature, pulse, blood pressure, and respirations) may or may not change as breathing continues and the heart keeps beating. At this stage, vital signs are not actually that vital, and they are monitored not for the patient but for the observers. There is no reason to obtain lab tests, which will look dire at this point and are not likely to provide any useful information. At this stage, family members should adopt the "care and comfort" goal and decline interventions that work against that goal.

Fever is not uncommon at the end of life, but it needs treatment only if there is associated discomfort. As oral intake decreases, kidney function declines, and then urinary output diminishes.

At this point, family members may revisit the question of IV hydration: "How can we let Mom die of dehydration?" It is important to remember that dehydration is part of the dying process. It is the effect of advanced disease, and as such is an expected and adaptive response of the body. In fact, the addition of IV fluids will only stress the heart and will likely result in the fluids ending up in the wrong places, such as in the lungs or any "low spots" (feet, backside, or hands depending upon positioning); this will only worsen the discomfort.

An analogy of this is the effect of a hard rain on parched August ground. The water just floods and pools and then flows away; it does not go to the places that need it. It does not cause any real improvement. As such, IV hydration for the actively dying person is an example of one way to prolong death—not to prolong life. It results in decreasing comfort rather than promoting it.

End of life, as natural as it is, can be an uncomfortable time for ancient ones due to pain, shortness of breath, nausea, profound depression, anxiety, or agitation. Suffering can have physical causes or be rooted in mental anguish. There are many medications available to keep the plan of comfort a reality. Caregivers need to watch for nonverbal manifestations of discomfort, such as moaning, grimacing, increased or labored respirations, or agitated restlessness; all are indications for medication. Compassionate healthcare providers support the use of frequent and liberal medications to promote comfort in this last stage of life.

Unfortunately, many of the medicines to promote comfort also result in side effects, and there can be tradeoffs with these interventions. For example, lack of appetite, constipation, confusion, and sedation are often consequences of effective pain relief. Other medications are often needed to counter these side effects.

Medicines should be given in response to individual needs. Often these medicines start out on an as-needed basis but then are scheduled every few hours to mitigate suffering in advance of these predictable situations of repositioning and personal care. There are often combinations of scheduled and as-needed medications. Relief may be quick and easy or it may require more time and trials to get unpleasant problems under control.

The Final Moments

When terminal decline has finally arrived, this should be a peaceful time, at least for the ancient one lying in bed. When a general mood of comfort is created, the effects are obvious and significant. I can tell how things are going with the patient by talking to the family, even before going into the room. When the family remains supportive and calm, the patient usually reflects those moods also.

The aim for a positive end-of-life experience is to keep the ancient ones comfortable enough so that their facial expression and body positioning are relaxed and calm and breath is easy. Aside from the medical interventions described earlier, simple measures based upon individual preferences and cultural traditions can provide a great deal of comfort. While some ancient ones may want hushed voices, dim lights, prayers, and classical or religious music, other times family chatter and normal conversation may seem more natural. It is even okay for children to be present if the circumstances allow. Many of these interventions are therapeutic to everyone in the environment and not just the patient.

When things are going well (and yes, a death can go well), loved ones and visitors often say things like, "At least he is comfortable." The sadness and grief cannot be minimized, but a peaceful death will give rise to calm witnesses.

As I've noted, family members need to be gently educated—and often reminded again—about the dying process, and they need to pace themselves physically and emotionally. It is very difficult to predict the duration of this last stage of life. It may last days or even weeks. Family and friends may set up a vigil at the bedside waiting for the end to come. They may assemble en mass, or they may rotate shifts. They may stay for hours or days. In any case, the living need food, drink, sleep, sunlight, and air.

Just as flight attendants tell passengers that in the event of an emergency they must put on their own oxygen mask before they can help anyone else, families must remember to take care of their own needs during this stressful period. This is particularly true for the equally elderly spouses, who are highly vulnerable at this time.

Family members and friends can take turns at the bedside, so that each can go home, rest, shower, and change clothes. Depending on the facility, it may be possible to arrange for food and drinks to be sent from the kitchen to ensure that everyone has a chance to get something to eat. Requesting additional chairs is another step family members can take to make sure everyone is comfortable.

* * *

Dying individuals should have the utmost dignity in their care. Attentive and gentle nursing care should keep the ancient ones clean, dry, comfortable, and well positioned. Patients who are unconscious should be spoken to as if present, touched as if awake, and cared for with as much kindness as possible.

The inevitability of death as the time draws near is an emotional time for everyone involved. Communication within the family and among the healthcare team is critical in providing this final, harmonious experience.

A Few Last Words

MANY RECENT TRENDS in the medical landscape have given me cause for optimism about the prospects for gentle care. There is more discussion about palliative care in both the medical and popular literature. With the aging of the baby boomers, we can expect the status quo to shift and provide more options that focus on the quality of life. As much as that generation did for the natural childbirth movement, we can hope to see similar acceptance of individualized approaches to advanced age and peaceful end-of-life care.

Today's ancient ones grew up in a very different world than the one that exists today. Many have seen the death of spouses, children, and countless friends, as well as suffering the loss of their independent lifestyles and often their own functioning bodies. It's a complicated experience to interact with these oh-so-old patients. People sometimes feel enormously saddened by exposure to these ancient ones.

It is important to remember, however, that these frail elders did not get to this point in their lives by being frail. They have lived through depressions, wars, and major social changes, and they have survived it all. The vast majority of them are tough, filled with an immense life force that has enabled them to thrive for so long. In order to have reached such an advanced age, they have demonstrated some almost superhuman strength of will and spirit.

In the fix-and-cure world of modern medicine, many practitioners struggle to recognize the professional rewards of caring for the ancient ones. Providers who feel obligated to try to treat these patients with a business-as-usual approach to their medical care often frustrate both themselves and their patients. However, when there is a solid and realistic plan of care in place that emphasizes the unique needs of the specific ancient one, it can be very gratifying to participate in the health care to promote independent functioning, ease suffering, and prevent medical futility.

As we look to the future, it is essential to recognize that these ancient ones deserve the best of care by providers who understand their goals. Family, friends, and healthcare teams must be valued, supported, and educated as we work together to honor the value and unique needs of these patients. It is essential to support and sustain the elders' health and independence for as long as possible. We must be able to allow for autonomy in decision-making, as their capacity allows, and encourage advance directives to guide their healthcare decisions on the last leg of a very long journey. And when the end of life comes, we need to see them out of this world with the kindness and compassion that everyone so deserves.

Glossary

active dying The end stage of life when the dying process has reached the point when there is no oral intake, very diminished alertness, and irregular respirations.

activities of daily living or **ADLs** A functional term referring to bathing, dressing, toileting, meal preparation, and self- feeding.

acute illness A new problem that presents itself and is expected to be resolved.

adaptive equipment Any device to assist with activities of daily living (ADL), such as reachers, specialized utensils for dressing or eating, or furniture modifications.

advance directives The formal guidance provided by a person in the event of his or her incapacitation. It includes the designation of a health care agent and wishes related to life sustaining treatments such as CPR, intubation, and mechanical intubation.

agitation The state of restless anxiety. Common in dementia.

ambulation Walking.

analgesic Medication used to ease pain.

anorexia A symptom referring to lack of appetite.

anticoagulant A medication affecting the blood's tendency to clot, used in the prevention and treatment of blood clots, aiming to protect vital organs from damage.

anxiety A common symptom of a sense of worry or restlessness.

aphasia A neurological disorder of communication, resulting in either difficulty speaking (expressive aphasia) or understanding language (receptive aphasia).

apnea Technically, absence of breathing. This occurs in intervals during sleep in some individuals and also during the phase at end of life called *active dying*.

appetite The description of one's interest in food and habits of eating.

aspiration A medical condition when food or fluids go into the lungs rather than the stomach, usually associated with cough, runny nose, tearing eyes, and "wet" voice. Commonly referred to as "going down the wrong pipe."

auscultation The process of listening to the sounds within the body with a stethoscope.

biopsy A term to describe the evaluation of a specific tissue sample to identify a diagnosis, such as cancer.

blood pressure A "vital sign" measuring of force of circulating blood on the artery walls measured by device called a sphygmomanometer. Ideally under 140/90.

cane A mobility aid that is hand held single staff used for stability and balance when walking.

cardiac arrest The cessation of heartbeat; death ensues promptly without CPR. A medical emergency when unexpected or unplanned for.

cardiopulmonary resuscitation or **CPR** An emergency intervention to restore the pulse and respiration in a patient with neither. A life-sustaining treatment.

catheter Any kind of flexible tube inserted into the body to allow fluids to pass in or out of the body. For example a "Foley" catheter drains urine out of body, an Intravenous or IV catheter infuses fluids into a vein.

cerebrovascular accident or **CVA** Commonly called *stroke*. A medical condition caused by a blood clot or hemorrhage in the brain, resulting in brain damage and some sort of functional impairment.

certified nursing assistant or **CNA** Health care providers with basic training supervised by nurses providing personal care of patients such as bathing, toileting and dressing.

chemical restraint A medication used to subdue or sedate an agitated patient.

chief complaint A sign, symptom or concern that prompts a medical encounter.

chronic illness A medical condition that is to be managed over time but not cured.

colonization A medical condition when bacteria is present in a particular body part but is not causing symptoms and may not require treatment.

colonscopy A type of specific endoscopic exam where a scope is inserted into the rectum to directly visualize the colon.

combative A behavior of physical resistance including hitting, scratching and biting. Common in dementia.

comfort measures Medical and nursing interventions that promote comfort and minimize discomfort, rather than treating the cause of the problem.

concentrator A medical device that extracts the oxygen out of air for inhalation by a patient.

constipation A common problem of insufficient or infrequent bowel emptying often associated with hard or dry stool.

contractures A condition of one or more joint that has become fixed in a flexed position.

crutches Mobility aids that fit under each armpit and extend to ground, used individually or in pairs to decrease weight on legs. Rarely suitable for use in advanced age.

culture and sensitivity or **C&S** A laboratory procedure that takes a sample of body fluids and determines the exact bacteria present and the appropriate antibiotics to be used to treat the particular infection.

custodial care A type of care that primarily assists with activities of daily living: bathing, dressing, toileting, and eating.

decubitus ulcer or **bedsore** or **pressure sore** A medical condition of skin breakdown, resulting mainly from pressure but also poor nutrition and immobility.

dehydration A medical condition of insufficient bodily fluids, either because of too little intake or too much output or both.

delirium A medical condition of agitation, confusion, and unpredictable behaviors occurring in response to a medical condition, medication, or stressful situation. This has an unpredictable course and can range from mild to life-threatening.

depression A medical condition with persistent sense of gloom, sadness, hopelessness, apathy, or despair.

diabetic foot care The special care taken on a daily basis to prevent skin problems of the feet, including washing and inspection of the feet to check for cuts, blisters, or irritation.

dialysis A medical treatment using a specialized machine to filter waste products from the body to replace the function of failing kidneys. A life-sustaining treatment.

diarrhea A medical problem of frequent loose or watery stools that, if persistent, can deplete fluids from an elderly body fairly quickly.

diuretic Medication used to remove fluid from the body by increasing urination.

do not resuscitate or **DNR** A medical order mutually agreed upon by the patient and medical staff to withhold cardiopulmonary resuscitation (CPR), in the event of cardiac or respiratory arrest.

Doctor of Osteopathy or **DO** Health care provider with a high level of authority and training. Combining training of traditional medical school and physical manipulations, they practice and specialize just like MDs.

edema A physical sign of swelling in a body part, due to injury or illness.

embolus A blood clot that forms in one place in the body, travels through the circulation, and becomes lodged in a different body part.

endoscopy A general term for putting a tube into the body to directly visualize the body's interior; biopsies can be obtained.

failure to thrive or **the "dwindles"** The slow and progressive weakness with declines in both physical and cognitive status not attributed to a known medical diagnosis.

feeding tube Any tube that provides access to the stomach or small intestine, used for nourishment, hydration, and medication. Gastric or G-tubes are inserted into the stomach through the abdominal wall. Nasogastric or NG-tubes are inserted into the nose and threaded through the throat into the stomach.

fingerstick The procedure of poking the finger with a sharp lancet to obtain a drop of fresh blood; frequently used to determine blood sugar.

fluid overload A medical condition, with several causes, of fluid retention in the body, commonly the lower legs and/or lungs.

formal healthcare Medical and nursing care provided by qualified and paid providers.

furniture-walking A common practice in the elderly of using furniture as handholds for stability when walking.

gait belt A fabric belt used to provide assistance and stability for transfers or walking. It is placed around the elder's middle and held by an attendant.

glucometer A simple diagnostic tool for the management of diabetes. A drop of blood is placed on a test strip and then inserted into this handheld device, providing immediate results of blood sugar.

health care agent or **health care proxy** or **health care power of attorney.** All of these terms refer to the designated person to assume the medical decision-making role, in the event of incapacitation.

health care proxy A legal document identifying the person who will assume the decision-making role in the event of a patient's incapacitation.

health care proxy activation The process of invoking the proxy by identifying and declaring the incapacitation of the patient by a qualified medical person.

Health Insurance Portability and Accountability Act of 1996 or **HIPPA** A national standard of care. Among other things, it protects the patient's privacy related to health information.

hemorrhage A medical condition referring to a large amount of bleeding that can be visible or occurring inside the body.

hospice Both a philosophy and an organization dedicated to dignity and comfort at end of life.

hospital or **healthcare-acquired infection** A particular type of infection developed by a patient during the course of treatment. Often caused by stronger than usual germs, such as pneumonia or UTI.

hypoglycemia A medical condition of low blood sugar, with symptoms of confusion, from insufficient eating or too much diabetic medication.

hypothermia A lower than normal body temperature from exposure to cold.

intake and output or **I&O** The measurement of fluids taken into the body and the fluids (primarily urine) coming out of the body.

illness A deviation from desired health status.

imaging studies These include x-ray, CT scans, and MRIs. Diagnostic tests that show an image or picture of the physical structures of body parts.

immobilizers A medical device used to maintain a healing position of an injured limb.

informal healthcare Medical and nursing care provided by family or friends.

injections Medications that require a needle and syringe to administer it directly into the muscle or tissue under the skin.

intravenous or **IV** A route of administration for fluids and medication that goes directly into a vein.

intubation A medical procedure when a tube is inserted into the airway and the patient is then connected to a mechanical ventilator. This is done in respiratory failure or temporarily during some surgeries. A life-sustaining treatment.

laxative Medication used to prevent or treat constipation and promote bowel movements.

level of care Concept in health care delivery that refers to where patients receive their medical services. This is what guides discharge practices. A patient will be discharged from the hospital when the "level of care" no longer meets hospital criteria.

libido The term used to describe one's sex drive or interest in sexual activity; not necessarily absent in the elderly.

lifeline A medical device that is worn as a bracelet or necklace that has the capacity to summon help in case of sickness or mishap.

living will An advance directive stating one's preferences for life-sustaining treatments. Its use is for the event of patient incapacitation and questions of ongoing treatment, not in emergency situations.

licensed practical nurse or **LPN** A nurse who has completed a certification program. Usually works close to patients doing meds and treatments.

mechanical lift A mobility device used to lift a patient in and out of beds and wheelchairs when they are unable to do so. They may be electric or manual, on wheels at bedside, or ceiling mounted.

mechanical ventilation The process of moving air in and out of the lungs using a bedside machine called a *ventilator* or *breathing machine*. A life-sustaining treatment.

medical doctors or **MDs** Healthcare providers with a high level of authority and training. They have completed medical school, internships, and residency programs and can be a general practitioner, medical specialist, or surgeon.

medication compliance A reference to how accurately medication directions are followed.

mental status testing An evaluation of the components of memory, judgment, insight, and reasoning with specialized testing.

metered dose inhaler or **MDI** or **puffer** A convenient, pocket-sized, device that delivers aerosolized medication through a mouthpiece and acts directly on the lungs. This device can be difficult for the elderly to coordinate.

mid-level practitioners Health care providers including advance practice nurses (nurse practitioners, certified nurse midwives, and nurse anesthetists) and physician assistants. They have completed specialized programs, at least a master level of education, and are able to diagnose and prescribe medications.

mobility aids Medical devices such as walkers, canes, and wheelchairs; used to improve the safety of getting around.

nausea A symptom of unpleasant stomach distress, queasiness, or near-vomiting.

nebulizer A small electric device that aerosolizes medication for inhalation to treat lung disorders. This can be administered through a mouthpiece or face mask.

neuropathy A medical condition of nerve dysfunction resulting in loss of sensation or function, or causing pain in various body parts, often hands and feet.

noninvasive ventilation or **CPAP** and **BiPAP** A medical treatment to force air into the lungs through a snug face mask. This can be used at night for sleep apnea or in emergency treatment for some kinds of respiratory failure.

nursing home An older term for the skilled nursing facility.

one-on-one Term used to describe one caregiver assigned to one patient due to intensive care needs or during epiosdes of severe confusion and restlessness.

orthostatic hypotension A medical condition of blood pressure dropping to a dangerous level with position change from lying or sitting, to standing. This is a common cause of falls in the elderly.

osteoporosis A medical condition of weakened bones causing them to break easily.

over-the-counter medication or **OTC** A category of medication that is available in a store without a prescription.

oxygen The part of air needed by the body to live. It can be provided in concentrated form when illness limits normal breathing. This is done by *nasal cannula*, tubes that insert slightly into nostrils, or by face mask.

oygenation saturation or **O2 sat** The assessment of oxygen in the blood, measured in percentages using a device called an *oximeter*. Normal is around 95%.

pain A symptom of unpleasant sensations or discomfort, of varying intensity, with numerous words to describe, as well as nonverbal manifestations.

palliative care A medical speciality focusing on control of symptoms and quality of life issues rather than correcting the underlying disease process.

PCP Either *primary care physician* if a doctor, or *primary care provider* if a nurse practitioner or physician assistant. Health care providers who are responsible for the overall medical care of the patient, coordinating the specialist care and attending to the "whole person."

peri-care The activity of cleaning the areas soiled in toileting: the perineum or "private parts."

physical restraint A device, usually cloth, applied to wrists or trunk and fastened to a bed to restrict movement and/or allow medical treatments in a confused person.

pneumonia A medical condition of infection of one or both lungs.

primary nursing An institutional style of nursing when one nurse is responsible for all nursing care on a particular shift; more common in hospitals.

PRN A category of medications used on an "as needed" basis, usually for symptom management. Also used in the directions for these medications, such as "every four hours PRN pain."

psychosis A psychiatric disorder of abnormal thoughts, including delusions and/or hallucinations.

pulse A "vital sign" of the assessment of the heart *rate* and *rhythm*. The *rate* is the number of beats per minute. Normal rate is 60 to 90 beats per minute. The *rhythm* is the quality of the beat. Normal heart rhythm is regular. Both rate and rhythm are measured by feeling the effects of each heartbeat at certain spots on the body or by listening over the heart with a stethoscope.

registered nurse or **RN** A nurse who has completed a college level program with an associate or bachelor degree.

regularity Term used to describe the pattern of one's bowel movement habit.

resistant germs or **superbugs** Microorganisms that have become stronger, due to exposure to antibiotics, resulting in infections that are more difficult to treat.

respirations A "vital sign." The assessment of number of inhalations taken in one minute, measured by observation. Normal is 18 to 22 breaths per minute.

respiratory arrest The cessation of breathing for an indefinite period, death ensues promptly without CPR or intubation and mechanical ventilation. A medical emergency if unexpected or unplanned for.

respiratory failure A serious medical condition when the body either cannot get enough oxygen or get rid of carbon dioxide. It can be either acute, which is a medical emergency, or chronic, with a slower onset.

rollator A mobility aid that has four wheels, hand brakes, and a seat.

route of administration Describes the way a particular medication gets into the body (for example, by mouth, injected into a muscle or vein, or applied to the skin).

schedule of administration Description of the timing and frequency of medications, such as once daily, every twelve hours, or as needed.

shortness of breath or **dyspnea** Symptom of difficulty breathing.

sign An objective observation of a physical finding, such as swelling or redness.

silent aspiration A medical condition when food or fluids enter the lungs without the usual associated signs and symptoms of cough, running nose, tearing, and "wet" voice.

skilled care Type of health care that requires the specialized skills of a doctor, nurse, or therapist. Each healthcare setting will have specific skill sets appropriate to their setting.

skilled nursing facility A healthcare facility that provides medical, nursing, and rehabilitation services to patients who do not require a hospital level of care, but are not well enough to go home. These facilities provide both skilled and custodial care.

sling A medical device used to hold an injured arm in a healing position.

suctioning The removal of respiratory secretions from the throat or mouth with a small vacuum tube.

sundowning A mental-status change of increased confusion and often agitation, in the afternoon and evening. Common in dementia.

suppositories Medications that are easily inserted into the rectum or vagina by putting them in as far as a gloved finger can reach.

symptoms The subjective perception of illness. Focal symptoms are specific and directly relate to the problem, such as pain or shortness of breath. Constitutional symptoms are generalized complaints, such as fatigue, weakness ,or malaise, and are less direct in the evaluation.

team nursing An institutional style of nursing when all the tasks for a patient are divided among several staff nursing members; more common in rehabs and skilled nursing facilities.

temperature A "vital sign" that is a measurement of body warmth, in degrees, using a thermometer. Normal is 98.6° F or 37°C.

thrombus A blood clot that forms in the body and stays in place, preventing normal circulation.

topical medication A medication that is applied on the skin either for direct action on the skin or to be absorbed for a systemic or whole-body effect. Also called *transdermal*.

tracheostomy A hole surgically created in the neck, used in medical conditions when there is an obstruction to breathing or for long-term mechanical ventilation.

transfers The functional process of moving from one surface to another, such as from bed to chair or wheelchair to toilet.

transient ischemic attack or **TIA** A medical condition of stroke-like symptoms (such as loss of function of body part or difficulty speaking) that resolve in less than twenty-four hours, sometimes called a mini-stroke.

tube feeding The process of instilling liquid nourishment through a tube to sustain life or supplement oral intake.

types of dementia Alzheimer's disease, vascular or multi-infarct dementia, metabolic encephalopathy, senile dementia.

urinalysis A simple diagnostic test of urine. A dipstick is used, results are immediately known, and it provides some information about bodily functions.

urinary tract infection or **UTI** A common medical problem of infection of bladder or kidneys that can have focal or constitutional symptoms.

vital signs A standard initial assessment of a patient, including temperature, pulse, respirations, and blood pressure.

walker A mobility aid that is a standing, four-legged frame. It is held with both hands, used to provide walking stability. It may or may not have front wheels, and can be modified or accessorized for personal needs.

weight-bearing status Description of restriction of pressure allowed on an injured limb (for example, non-weight-bearing means no weight at all on the limb).

Resources

Organizations and Services

Administration on Aging, Administration of Community Living. Part of the Department of Health and Human Services, this administration provides a profile of older Americans through an annual report, including data on the older population's future growth and general demographics.
www.aoa.acl.gov

AgingCare.com focuses on helping your loved one remain at home. It includes a caregiver forum and information on the daily challenges of home care.
www.agingcare.com

Alzheimer's Association serves as a comprehensive reference for all things Alzheimer's, including a 24/7 help line.
800-272-3900; www.alz.org

American Geriatric Society Health in Aging Foundation covers a broad range of topics, with an extra focus on medications.
www.healthinaging.org

American Health Care Association Quality Report. This site offers national information that is updated annually about skilled nursing facilities and trends in quality measures.
www.ahcancal.org/qualityreport

Argentum, which is a national trade association of professionally managed, resident-centered senior living communities, covers the many issues involved with this housing option.
www.alfa.org

Compassion & Choices. This group focuses on end-of-life options, offers a toolkit, and has a telephone support line.
800-247-7421; www.compassionandchoices.org

Eldercare Locator. This is a public service of the U.S. Administration on Aging to connect seniors with local community services.
800-677-1116; www.eldercare.gov

Family Caregiver Alliance offers a wealth of information about health conditions and caregiver strategies.

www.caregiver.org

HelpGuide.org provides a guide to mental health, with excellent housing option, elder abuse, and palliative care information.

www.helpguide.org.

Hospicenet. This is a service for patients and families facing life-threatening illness; it provides information for patients, families, and caregivers.

www.hospicenet.org

Medscape describes various medical conditions and treatments, including specific medication details.

www.medscape.com

National Center on Elder Abuse, Administration on Aging, Department of Health and Human Services. This organization provides a wealth of information on the many kinds of elder abuse.

www.ncea.aoa.gov

National Institute on Aging, branch of National Institute on Aging. This institute addresses research and advances in the science of aging and has up-to-date information on many issues related to aging.

www.nia.nih.gov

NIH Senior Health. This site offers health and wellness information for older adults from the National Institutes of Health.

www.nihseniorhealth.gov

Books

Chast, Roz. 2014. *Can't We Talk about Something More Pleasant?* A Memoir. New York: Bloomsbury USA.

Gwande, Atul. 2014. *Being Mortal: Medicine and What Matters in the End*. New York: Metropolitan Books.

Hartley, Carolyn P., and Peter Wong. 2015. *The Caregiver's Toolbox: Checklist, Forms, Resources, Mobile Apps and Straight Talk to Help You Provide Compassionate Care.* Boulder, CO: Taylor Trade Publishing.

Lebow, Grace, Barbara Kane, and Irwin Lebow. 2011. *Coping with Your Difficult Older Parent: A Guide for Stressed-Out Children.* New York: William Morrow.

Loe, Meika. 2013. *Aging Our Way: Independent Elders, Independent Lives.* New York: Oxford University Press.

Loverde, Joy. 2009. *The Complete Eldercare Planner, Revised and Updated Edition: Where to Start, Which Questions to Ask, and How to Find Help.* New York: Harmony.

Mace, Nancy L., and Peter Rabins. 2015. *The 36-Hour Day: A Family Guide to Caring for People Who Have Alzheimer's Disease, Related Dementias and Memory Loss*, Fifth Edition. Baltimore: John Hopkins University Press.

Manteau-Rao, Marguerite. 2016. *Caring for a Loved One with Dementia: A Mindfulness-Based Guide for Reducing Stress and Making the Best of Your Journey Together.* Oakland, CA: New Harbinger Publications.

McCullough, Dennis. 2009. *My Mother, Your Mother: Embracing "Slow Medicine," the Compassionate Approach to Caring for Your Aging Loved Ones.* New York: Harper Perennial.

Morris, Virginia. 2014. *How to Care for Aging Parents: A One-Step Resource for All Your Medical, Financial, Housing, and Emotional Issues*, Third Edition. New York: Workman Publishing Company.

Perkins-Carpenter, Betty, and Wes Fox. 1999. *How to Prevent Falls: Better Balance, Independence and Energy in 6 Simple Steps.* Penfield, NY: Senior Fitness Productions Inc.

Phelps, Rick, and Gary Joseph Leblanc. 2015. *While I Still Can . . . One Man's Journey Through Early Onset Alzheimer's Disease.* Bloomington, IN: Xlibris.

Volandes, Angelo E. 2015. *The Conversation: A Revolutionary Plan for End-of-Life Care.* New York: Bloomsbury.

Index